The Primordial Emotions

The Primordial Emotions:
The dawning of consciousness

Professor Derek Denton

Department of Physiology
University of Melbourne
Parkville 3010
Australia

Baker Heart Research Institute
Commercial Road
Melbourne 3004
Australia

Founding Director
Howard Florey Institute of Experimental Physiology
and Medicine
University of Melbourne

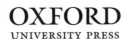

OXFORD
UNIVERSITY PRESS

OXFORD
UNIVERSITY PRESS

Great Clarendon Street, Oxford OX2 6DP

Oxford University Press is a department of the University of Oxford.
It furthers the University's objective of excellence in research, scholarship,
and education by publishing worldwide in

Oxford New York

Auckland Cape Town Dar es Salaam Hong Kong Karachi
Kuala Lumpur Madrid Melbourne Mexico City Nairobi
New Delhi Shanghai Taipei Toronto

With offices in

Argentina Austria Brazil Chile Czech Republic France Greece
Guatemala Hungary Italy Japan Poland Portugal Singapore
South Korea Switzerland Thailand Turkey Ukraine Vietnam

Oxford is a registered trade mark of Oxford University Press
in the UK and in certain other countries

Published in the United States
by Oxford University Press Inc., New York

© Éditions Flammarion, Paris, 2005
French title: Les Emotions primordiales et l'éveil de la conscience

The moral rights of the authors have been asserted
Database right Oxford University Press (maker)

First published 2005

British Library Cataloguing in Publication Data

Data available

Library of Congress Cataloguing in Publication Data

Denton, Derek A.
[Emotions primordiales et l'eveil de la conscience. English]
The Primordial Emotions: the dawning of consciousness/Derek Denton.
   Includes bibliographical references and index.
   ISBN-13: 978–0–19–920314–7
   ISBN-10: 0–19–920314–8
  1. Emotions.   2. Consciousness.   3. Mind and body.   I. Title.
[DNLM: 1. Consciousness—physiology.   2. Behavior, Animal—physiology.   3. Brain
Chemistry—physiology.   4. Emotions—physiology.   5. Instinct. WL 705 D415e 2006a]
   RC489.E45D46 2006   616'.08—dc22   2006008897

Typeset by Newgen Imaging Systems (P) Ltd., Chennai, India
Printed in Great Britain
on acid-free paper by Biddles Ltd., King's Lynn

ISBN-10: 0–19–920314–8 (Hbk)
ISBN-13: 978–0–19–920314–7 (Hbk)

10 9 8 7 6 5 4 3 2 1

Foreword

The theme of consciousness has been actively occupying theologians, philosophers and scientists for millennia. It raises endless disputes about its very nature and origins. I will always remember with emotion a seminar in Venice and a discussion with the distinguished Sir John Eccles, which almost ended in a burlesque fashion. The discussion was passionate and concerned the very substance of consciousness. He was on a vaporetto about to leave the shore while I was staying on the bank. Sir John suddenly grabbed my jacket, trying to convince me that consciousness does not have any materiality. At this very moment, the boat left the embankment: I only escaped the very material reality of a dive in the lagoon by a split second. At the basis of all the arguments about consciousness lies the entrenched assumption that men will never be able to understand this unique aspect of themselves which sets them apart from any other living creature of the planet. Science reaches its limits and they will not be breached. Objective knowledge clashes against a tangible unknown: *ignoramus ignorabimus*, wrote some eminent scientists of the end of the 19th century. Are we condemned to infinite ignorance!

This, of course, is not the case. The captivating book from Professor Derek Denton, world renowned specialist of animal instinct and integrative physiology, as can be expected, is diametrically opposed to this point of view. Even if Sigmund Freud in his *Fundamentals of Scientific Psychology* (which he did not publish) clearly positions himself as a physicalist, his work rapidly diverged from the brain biology of his time. Unfortunately this tradition continues today among the followers of his thought. Fortunately, since Freud, our understanding of the brain—neuroscience- has progressed dramatically from the point of view of the chemistry and genetics or biology of learning, but also from the viewpoint of cognitive functions and their physical workings, in particular with the spectacular advances in brain imagery. In the 1980s, the "Neuronal man", and then the "Astonishing Hypothesis" from Francis Crick, the publications of Gerald Edelman, have definitely established the scientific study of the neural basis of consciousness as empirically feasible and accessible theoretically and experimentally. Important research and thought have been dedicated to this topic since, such as the texts from Antonio Damasio, of Christof Koch, or "The Physiology of Truth". Derek Denton obviously lies within this trend of thought, but he goes further. To the question "What is the mind?" he tranquilly replies—the sentence is magnificent of simplicity- "what the brain does". But Derek Denton raises the fundamental question: we have to understand consciousness developed from the neuronal organization of the brain, as well as where it comes from and what are its origins? He differs radically from all his predecessors by taking a theoretical viewpoint which he demonstrates convincingly throughout the book. He has a unique expertise in areas of knowledge unfamiliar to those interested in consciousness: first, the experimental study of animal instinct, then an unequalled expertise about the physiology of water and salt. What relation can all of this have with consciousness?

According to Derek Denton, one should examine the early signs of consciousness, as they appear in the animal world and which are, according to him, "primordial emotions". Thirst, hunger, the need for air, for minerals, sexual desire are all necessary to the survival of living organisms. One cannot conceive life on Earth without feeding and reproduction. Those are commanding necessities. To satisfy them, there are particular neurobiological mechanisms pushing the organism to act promptly. Let us examine the example of thirst. It is caused by a sharp rise in sodium in the blood. In turn, it triggers the emotion of thirst, prompting the animal to drink. In three to four minutes of drinking, the organism is no longer thirsty: a gratification which ensures survival. Together with his collaborators, Derek Denton has demonstrated that the regions of the brain involved in this "consciousness" of thirst differ from those which control the level of sodium in the blood. For Derek Denton, the role of those gratification processes in evolution constitutes a major asset leading to consciousness in higher organisms. One may add, that when the animals feel this type of primordial emotion the source of water, food, or the sexual partner are not usually accessible or available. To obtain them, time is required. Christof Koch suggests the occurrence of those *delays* between the sensory stimulus and the execution of the action, is a specific test—the Turing test- of consciousness in the animal. The numerous examples taken by Derek Denton, from insects to octopus and fish, up to superior vertebrates, point in this direction. But it becomes clear, reading striking instances from the animal world, that a delay only is not enough to understand how consciousness is built. The organism needs to do more: it needs to use these delays to create a strategy, a plan of action : it needs to *organize* a behaviour, so that it can successfully answer to the primordial emotions that it feels inside. I will come back to this. Therefore a first minimum test for animal consciousness is, I propose, "delays plus the choice of a strategy".

Derek Denton, then, confronts his position with that formulated by the eminent scientist Gerald Edelman, according to which the first sign of consciousness would be the formation of an inner "scene" in which would develop representations, for instance visual, of the external world. Strongly opposing this viewpoint, Derek Denton proposes a major distinction. One needs to differentiate the perception of primordial emotions by internal receptors called interoceptive—which constitute a sort of initial "self"— from the perception of signals from the external world, for example visual, by exteroceptive receptors, such as the eye, directed to the outside. He reaches the definition offered at the beginning of the century by Brentano, of self-consciousness as the capacity to differentiate between one's own thoughts and that from the sensory information from the outside world.

This distinction illustrates straight away the original contribution of Derek Denton. First he examines those issues with animals: do bees have a collective consciousness? Can fish suffer? What is the difference between the conscious-ness of a squid and that of a mammal? Rigorous observations follow, stimulat-ing our curiosity. What is the reaction of a chimpanzee in front of a distorting mirror? Why did elephants from Mount Elgon in Kenya start mining a cave in the mountain up to the point of eroding their tusks, however necessary they are for their survival, in order to break the stones and extract salt from them? Derek Denton offers a precise and detailed analysis of those behaviours and underlines the numerous facts supporting his assertion. He demonstrates the central role played by primordial emotions, such as the hunger for salt in the elephants of Mount Elgon, combined with the occurrence of a primitive representation of oneself, as for the chimpanzee, which are sufficient to control both the innate and intentional actions.

The demonstration then follows at a more integrated level, and more "physical", so to speak. The reader reaches the privilege of being informed, with great clarity, of the most recent works of brain imagery on the theme of primordial emotions, in which Derek Denton was directly involved. The reader should prepare for a change of style. But he will appreciate to under-stand in detail how the experiment is conducted, how the materiality of our mental states is captured. What happens in our brain when we have the conscious sensation of thirst, when we drink water and thirst is quenched? Are the same areas activated when we are hungry or after we have eaten? What about the orgasm, this state of consciousness so constantly sought after by the whole of mankind?... These are essential questions for which a curious reader will find an answer in Derek Denton's lines!

The conclusion from these works in imagery, however preliminary, is already very edifying. Primordial emotions require, as expected, the oldest areas from the base of our brain: the medulla, the midbrain, the hypothala-mus, as well as the limbic system with the cingulate cortex, parahippocampus, the insula and the claustrum. Consciousness rises in the history of species with the differentiation of the primordial emotions. This internal awakening may have happened several times throughout evolution as for example with squid or with vertebrates. But it is not enough on its own to understand the behavioural consequences of that consciousness.

Derek Denton quotes a remarkable observation that enlightens us. A dehydrated frog is placed a few centimetres away from water; but unless by luck, it does not find the water and lets itself die. A lizard placed in the same conditions, on the contrary, searches for the water, finds it and drinks. The strategies of exploration designed by a small mammal are even more developed than those of the lizard. However, the neural structures used in primordial emotions evolved very little during the course of evolution. This is not the case of the cerebral cortex enveloping those old structures and developing very rapidly in vertebrates, from reptiles to man. Derek Denton then completes the question of conscious motivation with that of the exploration of the world, of the *plan* of actions to follow. The search for water requires multiple pieces of knowledge that the animal needs to integrate in order to drink: the map of the environment, the location of the water, the path to follow in order to reach it, one's own location with respect to the objective, the possible presence of predators to escape... The development of an integrating system, centralising, globalising these data, becomes indispensable.

The cerebral cortex plays this role. More precisely and with a great open mind, Derek Denton discusses the idea that Stanislas Dehaene and myself have proposed a while ago, of the contribution of long distance cortical connections which "link" the several cerebral areas concerned. This network, on a scale involving the whole brain, generates a work space in which a conscious planning of the behaviours to follow is created. At this stage, a new conceptual split must be introduced: the distinction between the "state" of this conscious work space and its "content", the collection of representations it creates. Let's first consider the state, or rather states, of the conscious space. Derek Denton adopts the point of view of the psychologist Baars and postulates that a system of neurons from the brainstem, rather archaic, called the ascending reticular formation, ensures access by the conscious space to sensory information, but also controls sleep and dreams. I compared this a few years ago to the console of a cortical organ selecting a particular keyboard particularly suited to the formation and treatment of specific mental objects. On the other hand, the content of the conscious space is different: it corresponds to the all-or-none mobilisation of groups of neurons distributed across the cortex, which implement the current perception of the external world—what may be called its knowledge, and the plan of action on the world, together with the primordial emotions.

As a conclusion, Derek Denton goes back to his initial assumptions. He shows how, in the human species, diverse and infinitely complex, primordial emotions play a central role in the states of consciousness: from the imperative access, almost totalitarian, of the conscious space, to the signals indicating the overfilling of the bladder or the distension of the rectum, up to the ever so subtle emotions raised by the meeting with a loved one or the appreciation of an art masterpiece. Re-assessing the proposals of Antonio Damasio on emotions, and comparing them to his own, Derek Denton brilliantly concludes his book with a theory, scientifically sound and pleasantly subtle, of the diversity of feelings and typically human emotions, often considered so mysterious.

A book of exceptional wealth, both deeply meaningful and constantly renewed, a book to read and reflect upon.

Jean-Pierre Changeux.

Acknowledgements

I am greatly indebted to Jean Pierre Changeux who has generously written a Preface to this book, and also to friends and colleagues who have kindly commented on specific chapters of this book, particularly John Blair-West, James Fitzsimons of Cambridge, Don Watson of Melbourne, and Peter Robb of Sydney, and Dr John McKenzie of Melbourne. I am also most appreciative of the discussions of issues raised in this book with Jean Pierre Changeux, Francis Crick, Roger Guillemin, Christof Koch, Peter Fox, Gary Egan, John McKenzie, Robert Naquet, Dame Miriam Rothschild and Sir Andrew Huxley. I am also most appreciative of discussion with Ann Butler and William Hodos on midbrain structures, and also of Dr Butler's reflections on the question of consciousness of pain in fish.

I am indebted to my colleagues involved in experiments on the neuroimaging of primal emotions. These include Dr Gary Egan, Professor Peter Fox, Dr.Robert Shade, Dr Lawrence Parsons, Dr Jack Lancaster, Professor Graeme Jackson, Dr Steve Brannan, Dr Mario Liotti, Dr Michael McKinley, Dr Robin McAllen, Dr John Johnson, Mr Frank Zamarripa, and Dr Michael Farrell. Dr Gary Egan, Ms Leonie Carabott, Mr Tim Silk, Dr Michael Farrell, and Ms Mariella McKinley generously helped with the illustrations. I am also indebted to Ms Lesley Walker who helped with the literature search and also prepared many of the diagrams, and Ms Sally Hood and Dr Michael McKinley for use of the NMR scans of their brains.

The experimental work in San Antonio, Texas and at the Howard Florey Institute and at the Brain Imaging Institute in Melbourne was supported by the Robert J. Jr. and Helen C. Kleberg Foundation, The G. Harold and Leila Y. Mathers Charitable Foundation, the Brown Foundation, The Search Foundation, and the Derek Denton Endowment Fund. I would also like to thank the Trustees of these Foundations for their help and encouragement. I am most grateful to Sir Evelyn de Rothschild for his generosity in providing Lodsbridge Mill as a tranquil setting in which to write, as was the case with my earlier books *The Hunger for Salt* and *The Pinnacle of Life*.

Lastly, my deep appreciation goes to Ms Eira Parry, my personal assistant, for the very large amount of patient work on the manuscript over 3–4 years, and for her suggestion bearing on the title of the book.

Contents

Permissions

I wish to thank Ian Redmond for permission to reproduce his photograph of elephants in the Kitum Cave, and also for the data he has generously provided on the behaviour of the elephants in the Mount Elgon Park. *The Journal of Physiology* (London) for permission to reproduce the fig. 1 from Denton 1956, Professor James Fitzsimons, and Cambridge University Press for use of segments of his table in his book *Physiology of Thirst and Sodium Appetite*. Dr Antonio Tataranni and colleagues for kindly preparing a figure on neuroimaging the state of hunger, which was derived from their data, and also for use of sections of fig. 1 from *Proceedings of the National Academy of Sciences USA*, **96**: 4569–4574, 1999. To Paul and Anne Kleinginna to use part of the table published in *Motivation and Emotion*, **5**: 345–379, 1981, and also Kluwer Academic/Plenum Publishers for their permission.

Oxford University Press to reproduce fig. 23 from *A Model of the Brain* by J.Z. Young (1964).

Dr Antonio Damasio and colleagues for permission to reproduce neuroimages from figs 1 and 2 of 'Subcortical and cortical brain activity during the feeling of self generated emotions', in *Nature Neuroscience*, **3**: 1049, 2000, and also to the Editor of *Nature Neuroscience*.

Dr Antonio Damasio for permission to quote from page 56 in *The Feeling of what Happens*, the section 'Emotions automatically divide organisms . . . . . . so is consciousness', and the publishers Heinemann, and the permission of Random House Group Ltd.

The American Academy of Arts and Sciences for permission to reprint portions of the table in the essay by George L. Gabor Miklos, 'The evolution and modification of brains and sensory systems', *Daedalus*, **127**(2): 197–216, Spring 1998.

Macmillan Publishers for permission to quote the passage 'As Descartes Le Monde . . . dualistic philosophy of man', from the article by Homer Smith in the *Historical Development of Physiological Thought*, Chandler McC Brooks and Paul Cranfield (eds), 1959.

The American Physiological Society for permission to reprint fig. 4 of 'Learning and other functions of the higher nervous centres' by F.K. Sanders and J. Z. Young, in the *Journal of Neurophysiology*, **3**: 501–525, 1940.

Dr R.B. Banzett and colleagues for permission to use neuroimages from fig. 5 of their paper in the *Journal of Neurophysiology*, **88**: 1500–1511, 2002, and the American Physiology Society, publishers of the journal.

Professor Gert Holstege and colleagues for permission to use neuroimages (figs 4–6, from their paper in *Brain* **120**: 111–121, 1997, and Oxford University Press. Figures 3 and 7 from their article published in the *Journal of Neuroscience*, **23**(27), 9185–9193, 2003, and the Society for Neuroscience, the publishers of *Journal of Neuroscience*.

Professor Per Roland and colleagues for permission to use their fig. 1 in *Science*, **271**: 512–515, 1996, and to the publishers of *Science*—American Association for the Advancement of Science.

Professor Bernard Baars for his permission to use fig. 1 of the paper he published jointly with the late Dr James Newman in *Concepts in Neuroscience*, **4**: 255–290, 1999.

Professor Jean Pierre Changeux for permission to use the fig. 11.1 from his book *L'homme de Vérité*, the Publishers, Odile Jacob Editions (Paris), and the National Academy of Sciences USA, this figure having appeared in *Proceedings of the National Academy of Sciences USA*, **95**(24), 14529–34, 1998.

Dr Ann Butler and Dr William Hodos for permission to use figures from *Comparative Vertebrate Neuroanatomy*, and to the publishers, Wiley-Liss Inc.

Professor R. Zatorre and Marelyn Jones-Gotman for permission to reproduce a neuroimage fig. I from *Brain Mapping*, A.V. Toga, and J.C. Mazziotta (eds), and the publishers Academic Press, a division of Harcourt Brace Ltd.

I am much indebted to Ms Mariella McKinley for drawing the figure of the two vases. Ms Genevieve Blair-West for the figure of sections of the brain, and Ms Lesley Walker and Ms Leonie Carrabott for preparation of several diagramatic illustrations.

List of Illustrations

Frontispiece
The approximate locality on a nuclear magnetic resonance (NMR) image of the brain of neuronal populations which subserve the genesis of some of the primal emotions. The neural correlates of the consciousness of the emotion do involve as well concurrent activation and deactivation in many other brain areas including the cerebral cortex and the reticular activating system of the midbrain.

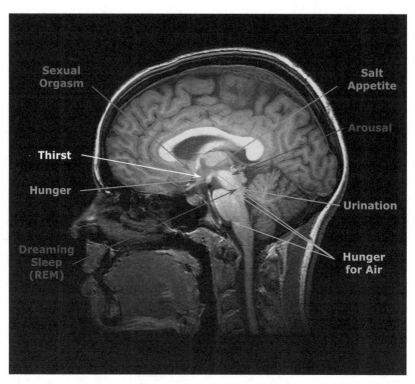

See also Colour Plate 16.

Part A

The hypothesis

Chapter 1

Introduction: The idea and context

To understand what is happening in the brain in the moment you decide, at will, to summon to consciousness a passage of Mozart's music, or you elect to take a deep breath, is like trying to catch a phantom by the tail. It is the essence of what Virginia Woolf said of 'thinking' in her essay on Montaigne. Reflecting on trying to describe what one is thinking to someone opposite, she says '... The phantom is through the mind and out the window before we can lay salt on its tail, or slowly sinking and returning to the profound darkness which it has lit up momentarily with a wandering light.'

The nub of this book is the issue of the first emergence in evolution of dim awareness—primary consciousness. Gerald Edelman, the distinguished Nobel Laureate, honoured for his contribution to immunology, has for a couple of decades addressed this problem. He directs the 'monastery of the mind', the Scripps Neurological Institute in La Jolla, San Diego, and has put forward his theory on the first emergence of consciousness—primary consciousness, as he calls it—in four books, which will be noted here in the text. It rests on the ability of the brain to 'create a scene'.

This book puts forward an alternative view to Edelman's. That is, that consciousness emerged in animal evolution as the primal or primordial emotions*, mostly driven by internal sensors (interoceptors). Primal emotion is defined as an imperious arousal compulsive of intention that has emerged during evolution because it is apt for the survival of the organism. Primal emotions, e.g. thirst, hunger, hunger for air, and pain, signal that the very existence of the creature is immediately threatened. The idea has been set out in a series of papers published in the *Proceedings of the National Academy of Sciences of the USA* from 1996 onwards, which, *inter alia*, deal with neuroimaging of primal emotions such as thirst and hunger for air.

Unravelling how the functions of nerve cells in the brain produce conscious awareness is arguably the greatest intellectual challenge in science today. The 'mind' is what the brain does. The debate and experimental data on this

---

* The terms "primordial" and "primal" are synonomous—meaning "existing at the very beginning"—Oxford Dictionary.

pivotal viewpoint ranges over territory as diverse as the memorable discussions between Elizabeth of Palatine and Descartes up to the striking implications of the experiments of Roger Sperry and colleagues on humans with a split brain. Here the brain was effectively split into two halves by surgically dividing the 200 million fibres of the corpus callosum that joins the two hemispheres. The patients had two separate minds.

One of the questions Elizabeth posed to Descartes was, 'if the soul possesses all the powers and habit of correct reasoning, how come these powers are so disturbed by an attack of the vapours?' This focuses attention on the fact that consciousness is determined by physical states of the brain, it being, for example, much upset by alcohol and hallucinogens. This is radically different from the idea that a separate mind perceives and acts through the brain. As Stephen Walker (1983) of University College, London says, it is much clearer that consciousness is determined by physical states of the brain than it is that a separate mind perceives and acts through the brain. Walker examines comprehensively these issues in an outstanding book *Animal Thought.*

Consciousness has emerged during the course of evolution because its advent gave great survival advantage. It has been honed on the anvil of natural selection. Nowadays, there is nothing novel about this idea. It is the overwhelming view of the majority of neuroscientists that the mind is what the brain does, and this is stated without ambiguity. Francis Crick with his friend James Watson, altered the course of human history by the discovery of the structure of DNA. It set in train the molecular biological revolution and genetic engineering. Over the past two decades or more Crick has addressed the issues of consciousness and brain function and concluded, as Lewis Caroll's Alice might have, that 'we're nothing but a pack of neurons' .... 'You, your joys and your sorrows, your memories and your ambitions, your sense of personal identity and free will, are in fact no more than the behaviour of a vast assembly of nerve cells and their associated molecules'. (Crick 1994).

This lucid statement in his introduction to *The Astonishing Hypothesis* (Crick, 1994) he sets in a relief to the Roman Catholic catechism:

Q: What is a soul?
A: The soul is a living being without a body, having reason and free will.

Gerald Edelman (1992) underpins his analysis of consciousness with a statement of his assumptions, including his insistence that 'the laws of physics are not violated . . . spirits and ghosts are out . . . I allow no spooks. Consciousness or mind is embodied.'

The distinguished British philosopher John Searle, (1997), now resident at the University of California, Berkeley, states, 'Brain processes cause consciousness but the consciousness they cause is not some extra substance or entity. It is just a higher level feature of the whole system'.

In setting out the ideas on primal emotion and the origin of consciousness, the endeavour will be to make the text understandable to a curious layperson. That is, to avoid technical jargon as far as possible, or at least, to try and explain such jargon if it is unavoidable in presenting the facts.

A primary aspiration of the book has been to set the key questions in a broad biological background. Thus, some material is novel, whereas other text aims to place these ideas in the context of present knowledge and viewpoint so as to give some overview.

We know that we are conscious because, among other things, we can distinguish between what thinking is going on in our own head, what we might wish to do, and what information is coming from the outside world. Consciousness has emerged with progressive brain development from primitive animals to humans because it carries a very high survival advantage. For an animal to be able to form images in the mind, and to choose an apt option for action in the light of appraisal of its immediate situation and its memory of past experience has great advantage. It may be much better than responding reflexly—that is, with an inflexible pattern that does not adapt according to the particular circumstances. It may make the difference between surviving or being killed. Survival allows it to hand on to its descendants the particular genetic structure that coded for the neuronal organization that subserved the propensity for conscious analysis of situations.

With regard to other members of our species, we can make a guess what they are thinking about, and see it confirmed by actions. Also we can ask. Language permits this, and what goes on in the mind can to an extent be described. There is a contrary view, that no one really knows that anyone else is conscious, a position that is called solipsism but nobody really believes it. However, when we come to animals, and the question of how to decide whether their behaviour reflects that they have conscious processes, simpler but like ours, there is the need to resort to means of deduction other than language. But Donald Griffin (1997), of Harvard University, who has led enquiry into the mind of animals, emphasizes animals can do a great deal to convey what is going on in their brain by behaviour and gestures, including vocalization.

Anticipating the more detailed analysis of the operational nature of concepts [Operational = performance of something of practical or mechanical nature (*Oxford Dictionary*)] we will recount further on, it can be noted here Bernard Baars (1988), in an influential book *A Cognitive Theory of Consciousness*, proposes one operational definition of consciousness. He asks the questions as to when any reasonable person would agree that someone just had an experience—that is objective evidence he/she saw a banana. They would be conscious of an event if, (1) they can say immediately afterwards that they were conscious of it, and (2) we can independently verify the accuracy of their report. That is, verifiable immediate conscious report is a very commonly used criterion. Baars indicates there are really four components in the operation as applied to the human: (1) consciousness of an event; (2) retrospective ability to direct conscious recall at will to the event; (3) the ability to recode (symbolize) the event into speech or gestures; and (4) the ability to voluntarily carry out those words or gestures.

Moving to the issue of animals, Griffin (1992) notes the philosopher Kenny's statement (1973) that one essence of mind is to have the capacity to operate symbols in such a way that it is one's own activity that makes them symbols, and confers meaning on them. Griffin takes the issue back to the renowned instance of symbolism inherent in the dances of honey bees—creatures with just under 1 million neurons. The bee's own activity makes her waggle dance a symbolic communication.

Perhaps this is seen at its best when the hive is swarming and seeking a new home. Scouts from a swarm who have visited cavities report distance, direction, and desirability to their sisters. The symbolic communication is far removed from the object it describes. Sometimes the waggle dance may refer to cavities or a food source the dancing bee has not visited for some hours. Essentially the search is for an ant free, dry, dark cavity, and the waggle dances by different bees convey the information on quality, the final decision reached being something of a group decision—a consensus that is not reached quickly.

The marking of individual dancers by the scientist Lindauer (1971), who made this study, also established that a bee that had espoused one cavity by its dance, then visited other cavities about which a sister bee had danced vigorously, and thereupon danced in favour of this new cavity rather than the one it had advocated earlier. In Griffin's view this communicative versatility suggests the bees are expressing simple thoughts.

Summary of the aim of this book

It is to consider the first emergence of primary awareness, that is primary consciousness, in the evolutionary process.

Gerald Edelman (1992) defines primary consciousness as the ability to construct an integrated mental scene in the present. It does not require language or a true sense of self. It is based on *perceptual categorization* of inflow from vision and other sensory information about the external world.

Perception is defined by Edelman as discrimination of a particular object or event through one or more of the senses. It depends on the ability to separate it from everything else picked up from the outside world by eyes, ears, and nose at any given instant in time.

Categorization, Edelman says, treats non-identical objects or events as equivalent. That is, a 'chair' is something in general terms that somebody sits upon, but it may have three legs, four legs, or two or three flat surfaces to the floor. Thus, perceptual categorization is the ability to carve up the world of signals (perception) into categories adaptive for a given species. This can be easily demonstrated in animals. Professor Herrenstein has experimented on the cognitive abilities of pigeons. Pigeons can pick out from dozens of photographs those with a human figure in them; whether it is an infant, a side face, someone with their back to the camera, naked or clothed, under a tree, and numerous other situations. If it pecks a picture with a human figure in it, it gets food. If no human is in the photograph, it does not. The pigeon gets it right about 80% of the time.

Edelman's is basically a *distance receptor theory* of the neurophysiological organization subserving the emergence of primary consciousness. Distance receptor means that it is based on information that comes in through sense organs that detect things at a distance—the eyes, ears, and nose.

I see the first emergence of consciousness differently.

I think the imperious states of arousal and compelling intentions to act that characterize *the primal emotions* were the origins of consciousness. The term 'primal' or primordial emotion is being used for the *subjective element* of instinctive behaviour, which subserves control of the vegetative systems of the body. The instinctive mechanisms are, of course, genetically programmed. The great Harvard psychologist, William James, stated in his landmark book *Principles of Psychology* (1890) published over a hundred years ago, the inexorable binding of emotion and instinct, it being a genetically determined structural relation. He says, 'In speaking of instincts, it has been impossible to keep them separate from the emotional excitements which go with them.' Further '. . .. That every object which excites an instinct excites an emotion.'

Primal emotions signalled that the very existence of the organism was threatened. Examples of primal emotion include thirst arising from dessication of the organism, or breathlessness or 'hunger for air', which occurs with choking or any other cause that cuts off the air supply. Such overwhelming sensations that commandeer the whole stream of consciousness are choreographed from the lower or basal areas of the brain. The initiating signals come from sensors monitoring and reacting to the physicochemical composition of the blood reaching the base of the brain. *The sensors concerned, which are inside the body, are called 'interoceptors'. This is in contrast to the 'exteroceptors'—the distance receptors.* They are the operations of what is termed the vegetative systems, which regulate and maintain the constancy of the internal environment of all the cells of the body.

A.D. Craig (2003) of Phoenix, Arizona, refers to pain as a homeostatic emotion reflecting an adverse condition in the body, such as thirst, hunger for air, or temperature deviation, which demands a behavioural response. (The term 'homeostasis' is used for the physiological processes that keep the conditions within the body constant.) In terms of an overview on this crucial issue of the utility of consciousnesss, William James (1890) stated 'the empirical connection between subjective feelings of pain and objective injury on the one hand, and between feelings of pleasure and life enhancing activities could only be explained if evolution had rendered subjective states effective in adapting animals to their environments. That is, if consciousness had not served some useful purpose it would not have evolved.'

What the interoceptors do in a way is to 'taste' (detect) change in, for example, the salt concentration of the blood reaching the brain, or the carbon dioxide content of it, or its temperature, or its sugar content and so on. Explicitly, if the salt concentration of the blood rises it causes thirst. By contrast, the opposite facet of this physiological control system is that in some species of animals, particularly the grass eaters, which represent the wild game and pastoral animals of the planet, if the salt concentration falls it sets in train an avid desire to seek and eat salt. The grass eaters are the species most likely to become salt deficient. The direct impact of the vast salt-deficient areas of the interior of continents and also the mountains of the planet falls on them.

Much of the nerve cell organization and their connections that subserve such vegetative primal emotions are hard wired. That is, the components are set in place and connected up by the action of genes during embryonic development. Thus with primal emotions it is a genetically determined neural organization in the evolutionary ancient basal brain. Examples of primal emotions other than those already instanced include hunger, pain, desire to sleep following deprivation, and sense of extreme temperature change including that of the core of the body, sexual orgasm, and the thwarting of visceral functions.

Thus, a large part of the organization of the vegetative systems with their interoceptor detectors is down, as it were, in the basement of the brain (in the medulla, midbrain, and hypothalamus) like the elemental processes of arousal and sleep themselves (frontispiece). By contrast the higher order activities of vision, hearing and cognitive processes are organized to a great extent in the grey matter of occipital, parietal, temporal and frontal lobes—the neocortex—the upper levels rather than the basement of the brain.

From this evolutionary viewpoint two big questions follow.

1 At what stage or stages in the evolution of animals did primary consciousness first emerge?

2 What kind of anatomical and functional organization of the brain emerged to subserve this primary consciousness as it appeared?

These are difficult but fascinating questions. They open a vast panorama of biology. The first question must and does centre on animal behaviour and how to interpret it at different levels of phylogenetic (evolutionary) development. The second is a matter of the neuroanatomical (brain structure) and neurophysiological (brain function) changes that occur with development of a more complex brain. This occurs progressively in the course of evolution—that is, ascent of the so-called phylogenetic (evolutionary) tree. Scientific advance in answering these questions has been dramatic over the last century. Our discussion will lead to brain imaging of consciousness during states of primal emotion such as thirst and hunger for air, body temperature change, sexual orgasm, and during emotions such as anger, fear, and hate, as well as with higher order cognitive and intellectual processes.

However, only portions of an enormous field can be covered in this book. Some issues not often covered during a discussion of consciousness are made central. This is perhaps reflected in the fact that the indexes of outstanding contemporary books in this field such as those of Edelman, Crick, Damasio, Penrose, and also LeDoux, contain little or nothing on issues such as thirst, hunger, hunger for air, mineral appetites, and rarely pain, or for that matter thwarted visceral functions such as the strong desire to pass urine. This latter interoceptor driven function is accompanied by sensations that may rise to the level of something so totalitarian that we might call it imperious, and, as most of us know, eventually by an experience akin to pain.

Dealing with the feelings associated with such distension of bladder or rectum, Jaak Panksepp (1998) of Bowling Green, in a book *Affective Neuroscience*, states that, 'Obviously several types of cognitive and emotional arousal occur in any strong motivational situation. Consider the simple cases of excessive bladder and rectal distension.' He goes on to say

> "feelings of distension can become incredibly insistent, filling our minds with nothing but the urge for relief. The feelings are so insistent that it is difficult to sustain other thoughts in one's mind. Unfortunately, we know little about the neural systems which subserve such feelings, but it is possible they are organized quite low in the brain stem level. If we could specify the exact neural systems that create such feelings we would probably understand more about consciousness than presently can be found in most of the learned texts on the topic."

In relation to thirst, and the application of the term 'primal emotion' to it, it is notable that in the most scholarly compendium of present knowledge on the subject of thirst, James Fitzsimons (1979) of Cambridge University, states, 'We might talk of the sensation of thirst when dehydration is moderate, but there is no question that severe dehydration produces a sensation so distressing that strong emotion is aroused by it'. Likewise Panksepp (1998), referring to respiratory distress or impairment of our rhythmic breathing, states that when such events occur a very powerful emotional state arises. He goes on to state that human 'panic attacks' may emerge in part from activation of this powerful emotional response system. The issue of the precise use of words in descriptions of affective states and intentions when the vegetative systems of the body, which have control centred in the hypothalamus, midbrain and hindbrain, are distorted from their normal dynamic equilibrium state will be addressed in Chapter 12. However, the essence of the approach adopted, and its relation to the view of William James has been set out above.

The majority of neuroscientists concerned with analysis of consciousness have set themselves a much loftier and challenging goal than the vegetative systems. Many have focused on visual awareness or other perception of the external world with all the cognitive and high order intellectual processes involved. Emotion has also been the centre of detailed analyses (e.g. the outstanding work of Antonio Damasio (1999(b)) and his group at Iowa), but not the primal emotions. These primal emotions contrast, in a relative way, with emotions such as anger, hate, love, and fear, which are largely set in action, for example, by inflow from the eyes and ears resulting in assessment of a situation; i.e. situational perception determined by the distance receptors ignites the emotion.

These emotions, such as anger, love, and hate, can be summoned at will to consciousness, and can then be neuroimaged. It is 'scenario-induced emotion'. However, it is highly questionable whether we can electively, at will, in the same way summon to consciousness the sense of experiencing the imperious sensation of thirst, hunger for air, hunger, or pain. These emotions are clearly organized differently in the brain.

It is also questionable whether it is possible at will consciously to experience a sexual orgasm—although aroused sexual desire can lead to the imagining of circumstances that could culminate in the event. Perhaps it would not be good for the survival of the species if it were easily possible. However, it is possible to experience orgasm when asleep during dreaming.

Of course, once the primary emotions have invaded the stream of consciousness in the higher animals, the processes of perceptual categorization and memory will enter the ring and come to bear on the intention of the animal seeking immediate gratification of the need, which is signalled by the powerful emotion. The past history of the organism will contribute to the choice of an apt option. So with progressive evolution, the two processes—primal emotion and perceptual categorization—will interlace and anneal with enormous natural selection advantage to the organisms.

The interesting question, however, is which came first. Or were they phylogenetically contemporaneous and then melded functionally at a very early stage? Edelman's view is that, along with control of movement, perceptual categorization is the most fundamental process of the vertebrate nervous system. This would seem a penetrating insight in relation to organization of brain development during evolution. However, there are grounds for thinking that perhaps the primal emotions came first. They are choreographed from the hard wired interoceptor systems of the basal brain where, as noted above, control of arousal of the organism—its actual awakening—and of sleep are also resident. The emergence of primal emotions as first consciousness involved a gradual evolution forwards (rostrally) of the structure of the brain. As a consequence of this, it is plausible that these hard wired systems of complex reflexes in the hypothalamus, midbrain, and hind brain melded via pathways with the giant relay system of the thalamus. Thereupon they melded with the earliest cortical elements that evolved. These early cortical structures are the so-called three- and five-layered allocortex and transitional cortex including the cingulate, parahippocampal, and insula regions. The higher association cortex, including, frontal parietal, temporal, and occipital lobes of later evolutionary development—the isocortex—has six layers of cells. As will be recounted, neuroimaging of the primal emotions reveals a functional organization in which the evolutionary ancient areas of the brain play a dominant role.

The scope of the book

To this point, the Introduction has presaged the main theme to be analysed in the book and aspects of it in physiological, and also psychological thought as exemplified by William James. However, description here of other ways the book is developed hopefully will be helpful to the reader in terms of explaining the connectivity of the ideas in it, and why certain sections are included.

In Chapter 2 there will first be consideration of how concepts arise in science. This is pertinent because of the great difficulty of definition in analysis of consciousness. The ideas of Nobel Laureate physicist P.W. Bridgman are central. Then, because of its intrinsic interest in any tract on consciousness, the issue of self-awareness, of being the object of one's own attention, will be discussed. Evidently it is a higher order function. The issue of how far down the phylogenetic tree it can be demonstrated bears on the general issue of continuity in the evolution of consciousness as stated by T.H. Huxley. In this regard it seems highly probable that perceptual awareness emerged long before any self-awareness.

In the same vein, though our primary theme is the primordial aspects of consciousness, in Chapter 3 the view has been taken that it is anything but tangential to recount the ideas of some distinguished scientists and philosophers on the general nature of conciousness. This brings in historic background, and perhaps as well, gives some generalized perspective for the reader against which the discussion of the more particular matter of this book is set.

Thereupon, in Chapter 4 the issue of consciousness in animals is addressed broadly in relation to experimental evidence at differing levels of the phylogenetic tree—e.g. squid, fish, snakes, and mice. In relation to affirmation of consciousness in animals, attention is drawn to data pertinent to the Turing test of consciousness as enunciated by Koch and Crick, and described in Christof Koch's recent outstanding book *The Quest for Consciousness*. Chapter 5 gives an account of the remarkable salt mining by elephants carried out in the dark, deep in Kitum Cave on Mt Elgon in Kenya. The behaviour suggests a cultural transmission of knowledge.

In Chapters 6 and 7 Edelman's and my theories of the emergence of consciousness in the evolutionary process are discussed. As consciousness of thirst is the exemplar we have used for the neuroimaging of primal emotion, a discussion of the basis and evolution of water control precedes the account of the neuroimaging studies. The lay reader may find some parts of Chapter 8 quite interesting general information, having been themselves thirsty and actually wondered how the consciousness of it arose. However, Chapter 8 might be bypassed, and the reader proceed straight to Chapter 9 on the neuroimaging of thirst. Chapter 10 provides data on the neuroimaging of several other primal emotions, and also the distance receptor evoked emotions involving situational perception such as with anger, or fear.

Chapter 11, as with Chapter 3 is an important part of the endeavour to give an overview of consciousness. It includes embodiment of the thoughts of Dehaene, Changeux, and Kerzberg, and those of Baars and Newman on the heirarchial organization of higher consciousness. A global neuronal workspace, as an integrating system is envisaged to be the operating high point. Processors for various crucial functions, such as perception or memory project to the workspace, with privileged access falling to some according to pertinence and past experience. Obviously, the primal emotions when imperiously occupying the stream of consciousness would have had privileged access to the workspace through perception processors.

The final chapter, Chapter 12, addresses the mystery of the nature of emotion. What actually happens in the circumstance of the welling up to consciousness of the raw and imperious sensations annealed with compelling intention is not well understood. Clearly there is an enormous range of emotions, and if the heirarchy were considered as a triangle, the primal emotions would be at the base, and the aesthetically engendered emotions such as the joy of listening to Bach, would be at the apex. There have been quite diverse ideas on what an emotion is and many of these are discussed, including those of Antonio Damasio.

Some sections of the text of the book will be printed in boxes as done here. Such sections may deal with brain anatomy, physiological mechanisms, or detailed argument. The general reader might pass them by without losing the gist of the argument of the book, but they may be worth considering by those with a background in science— particularly neuroscience. The issue arises mainly in chapters describing the results of neuroimaging of emotions, where a lot of anatomical details are recorded, but also in some sections on animal behaviour and the physiological basis of thirst

---

Chapter 2

The definition of consciousness, and self-awareness

When discussion of consciousness erupts in a scientific group, or for that matter, in any gathering, a likely early issue is—define the term! What is meant by consciousness? According to one's viewpoint, this is exceedingly difficult or reasonably straightforward.

Many basic facets of biology have been illuminated in the process of attempting definition. Some scholars aim to state what they see to be the essence. Others veer towards listing the elements they recognize to be embodied in having a stream of consciousness.

Gerald Edelman is fond of quoting William James (1890), Professor of Psychology at Harvard, who said of consciousness that it is something the meaning of which 'we know as long as no one asks us to define it . . . an accurate account of it is the most difficult of philosophic tasks.' James says consciousness 'does not appear to itself to be chopped up in bits. It is nothing jointed, it flows.' He says a 'river' or 'stream' are the metaphors by which it is most naturally described. In talking of it hereafter he says, let us call it 'a stream of thought, of consciousness, or of subjective life'. James adds further in his analysis of the stream of thought that 'it is always interested more in one part of its object than in another, and welcomes and rejects, or chooses all the while it thinks.' Selective attention and deliberative will are patent examples of this choosing activity. There is a final point of James' analysis to mention here. He reflects that the human race as a whole largely agrees as to what it shall notice and name and what not. However, there is one extraordinary case in which no two people ever are known to choose alike. One great splitting of the whole universe into two halves is made by each of us. However, James says, we all draw the line of division between them in a different place. That is, we all call the two halves by the same names and those names are 'me' and 'not-me' respectively. He adds that the altogether unique kind of interest that each human mind feels in those parts of creation that it can call 'me' or 'mine' may be a moral riddle but it is a fundamental psychological fact!

J.Z. Young, the great British zoologist and neuroscientist, agrees with the Viennese philosopher, Brentano in emphasizing that beings having conscious intentions can recognize a difference between their own thoughts and the sensory information coming in from outside. This implies self-consciousness. Young quotes Searle's (1984) position, 'the second tractable feature of mind is what philosophers and psychologists call intentionality, the feature by which our mental states are directed at, or about, or refer to, or are of objects or states of affairs in the world other than themselves.'

Young stresses a key issue. It is crucial to reiterate it. *Intentionality is a property of mental life that may refer to entities that are not observable at the time.* Thus, intentional thoughts may be different from other purposive thoughts where the aim is clearly in view. The brain can be a repository of expectations garnered and deduced from earlier experience. Such a body of desire and intention may, as we have said, be set in train by chemical changes within the animal. These fire off interoceptors that cause consciousness of thirst, as in the case of rise of blood salt concentration. Based on a portfolio of memories including the geography of its situation, an animal may develop a strong intention to seek a water hole where it remembers it saw water when passing and did not need water. Or it may remember where it drank water earlier on. It is different to feeling thirsty and simply having the sight of water actually in front of the eyes.

For perspective, it needs to be remarked at this point that it is obvious what is being talked about in the case of thirst is in the basement of conscious experience. At a much higher level, there are phenomena of intuitive insight and genius. Don Watson points out how Freud refused to believe Shakespeare could divine the psychology of Hamlet without parallel experience. However, with writing, painting, and dance, the individual genius seems to uncover realities of consciousness we did not know existed. Indeed, it is in the experience of individual creative people that often it would appear that what comes up as a flash of intuitive insight has been thought about for some time, and the solution suddenly pops up. A classic example would be the solution to mathematical problems. This is discussed in the book recording the debate between Jean Pierre Changeux, of the College de France, and Alain Connes, the distinguished French mathematician (*Conversations on Mind, Matter and Mathematics*, 1995).

The thoughts of James and Young noted above, voiced some time ago, can serve as the overture to views I wish to recount of some other contemporary neuroscientists, apropos definition of consciousness. I will outline also in this chapter a brief consideration of the important subject of the nature of concepts in science as analysed by P.W. Bridgman.

Francis Crick in his book *The Astonishing Hypothesis* (1990) says, 'Consciousness is a subject about which there is little consensus, even as to what the problem is . . . Everyone has a rough idea of what is meant by consciousness. It is better to avoid a precise definition of consciousness because of the dangers of premature definition which might be misleading, or overreactive, or both.' Parenthically he adds 'If anyone thinks this is cheating, try defining for me the word 'gene'. So much is now known about genes that any simple definition is likely to be inadequate. Thus, how much more difficult to define a biological term when rather little is known about it.'

Crick poses a key question, 'It seems probable at any one moment some active neural processes in your head correlates with consciousness, while others do not. What are the differences between them?'

It is entertaining and diverting that 150 years earlier, a man whom like Crick and his friend Jim Watson also changed the course of human history, was considering the definition of what was, in effect, genetically determined behaviour. Charles Darwin wrote at the beginning of the chapter on Instinct in *Origin of Species* that he would not attempt to define instinct—but then to an extent went on to do exactly that. He noted that many instincts are so 'wonderful' that his readers would have, he said, probably had in mind that their development was a difficulty sufficient to overthrow his whole theory. He said

> I will not attempt any definition of instinct. It would be easy to show that several distinct mental actions are commonly embraced by this term; but everyone understands what is meant when it is said that instinct compels the cuckoo to migrate and to lay her eggs in other birds nests. An action which we ourselves require experience to enable us to perform when performed by an animal more especially a very young one, without experience, and when performed by many individuals in the same way, without their knowing for what purpose it is performed, is usually said to be instinctive. But I could show that none of these characters are universal. A little dose of judgement or reason, as Pierre Huber expresses it, often comes into play, even with animals low on the scale of nature.

At this point it is perhaps useful to consider how concepts may be defined.

Bridgman and concepts

The meaning or definition of a concept was analysed comprehensively by the physicist, P.W. Bridgman in his book *The Logic of Modern Physics* (1927). He proposes that the content of a concept, the basis of physical knowledge, lies in a series of operations. He illustrates this operational attitude to a concept by examining *length*, and deals with measuring, say, a house. As a rough description one starts with a measuring rod. One lays it on the object so one end of it coincides with one end of the object, marks on the object the position of the other end of the rod, and then moves the rod along in a straight line extension of its previous position until the first end coincides with the previous position of the second end. The process is then repeated as often as we can and *the length* is called the total number of times the rod was applied—how many rods long. He notes this apparently simple procedure is exceedingly complicated. For example, one needs to be certain the rod is at the standard temperature its length is defined, or make a correction for it. Correction would be made for gravitational distortion of the rod if a vertical length is measured. It is necessary to be sure that the rod is not a magnet or subject to electrical forces. These precautions would occur to every physicist.

In principle, the operations by which length is measured should be precisely stated. This is complicated enough for stationary bodies. Bridgman (1927) says, when it comes to the operation of measuring the length of a very large object such as, in the first instance a large tract of land, the operation uses a surveyor's theodolite. This involves extending over the surface of the land a system of co-ordinates starting from a baseline measured with a tape in a conventional way. Sightings are made on distant points from the extremities of the line. The angles are measured. He says one essential change has occurred. The angles between lines connecting distant points are now angles between beams of light. It is assumed light travels in a straight line. Thus, in extending the system of triangulation over the surface of the earth the geometry of the light beams is Euclidean. In checking this assumption, Michelson's experiments showed the direction the beam of light travelled around the triangle with respect to the rotation of the earth affected the result. *Bridgman's point is that the concept of length has undergone a very essential change of character even within the range of terrestrial measurements.* A tactual concept has been substituted for by an optical concept, complicated by an assumption about the nature of our geometry.

He points out that the procedure is entirely optical when the extension is made to solar and stellar space. If it is desired to measure the length of bodies moving with high velocities such as are found in nature, it is necessary to adopt another definition. Other operations are used for measuring length. This is what Einstein did. Bridgman says that as Einstein's operations were different from the operations above, his length does not mean the same as our length. The observer who is to measure the length of a moving object must first extend over his entire plane of reference a system of time co-ordinates. At each point of his plane of reference there must be a clock. All these clocks must be synchronized.

Without tracking further Bridgman's analysis of stellar and subatomic measurements of length in relation to the operation involved, it is conspicuous that in principle he thinks that by changing the operations we have really changed the concept. Therefore, to use the same name for these different concepts over the entire range is dictated only by considerations of convenience. He says that these may sometimes prove to have been purchased at too high a price in terms of lack of ambiguity. Bridgman says, that because two different sets of operations that give the same results in a certain context may result in something 'measurably different' in a completely different context 'it is necessary to be aware of joints in conceptual structure'.

The nature of concepts, according to the operational point of view, is the same as the nature of experimental knowledge, which is often hazy. Almost all physical experience is buried in the discovery of the operations that may be usefully employed in describing nature. If a specific question has meaning, it must be possible to find operations by which an answer may be given to it. In summary, Bridgman (1927) says we should not permit ourselves to use conceptual tools of which we cannot give an adequate account in terms of operations. Here I have only briefly touched upon Bridgman's use of length to illustrate his argument.

He points out that discovery of the number obtained by counting the number of times a stick of arbitary length could be applied to objects and could be simply used to describe them, was one of the most important and fundamental discoveries ever made by Homo sapiens.

The concept of self-awareness and an operational definition of it

An instance where this discipline of concept analysis in physics might be relevant to our field of enquiry is in the matter of *self-awareness*. This is the highest form of awareness variously described as the inward turning of consciousness, being the object of one's own attention, contemplation of one's own existence, reflective awareness, being conscious of being conscious, or as Shakespeare had Hamlet's mother say 'O Hamlet! Speak no more; Thou turnst mine eyes into my very soul; and there I see much black and grained spots as will not leave their tinct.'

Language makes it possible for members of the human species to believe without doubt that their fellows are conscious and self-aware. However, when it comes to animals lower in the evolutionary scale, which are without language, the issue is whether there is an operational basis of measuring 'self-awareness'.

Self-awareness in apes: mirror self-recognition and effect of 'circus' distorting mirrors

Dr Gordon Gallup (1970, 1975, 1978, 1991) has pioneered work in this field on the basis of mirror self-recognition.

Many species of animals when confronted with their reflection in a mirror react as if to another member of the same species and engage in aggressive display. This is seen in animals as varied as fish, birds, sea lions, and primates. A bird may fight its image in a window or hub cap to exhaustion. Similarly, human infants may react to their reflection in a mirror in the same way as they would to another infant. They endeavour to embrace and kiss the reflection— a new playmate! As is the case with animals, infants may reach behind the mirror to search for the other individual. At about 18 months of age, the behaviour of the human infant in the face of its mirror reflection becomes self-directed. It examines itself with the aid of the mirror. The verbal indications of a stable self-concept with use of self-reference pronouns (me) or the individual's name usually do not appear until about 2 years of age.

In terms of what we might regard as an operational definition of this concept—self-awareness—Dr Gallup conducted some ingenious and now very well known experiments.

He studied four pre-adolescent male and female wild born chimpanzees that were reared as a group. Each was put by itself for 8 hours a day in a room empty except for a mirror placed in front of the cage. Over a period of 10 days a clear-cut behaviour change occurred. At first each of them responded like they would to a rival. They bobbed, vocalized, and threatened. By 3 days this ceased. After 4 days behaviour was exclusively self-directed. The mirror was used for access to otherwise inaccessible information. Food was picked from between the teeth. Visually guided manipulation of the anogenital region occurred. Bubbles were blown, and faces were made. Corners of lips were turned back to see into the mouth. The chimpanzees clearly recognized the identity of the reflection.

To more rigorously define the behaviour, the chimps were anaesthetized. While unconscious, an odourless red dye was painted over the eyebrow or on top of the ear—positions impossible for the animal to see without a mirror. A careful score of the animals spontaneous or random touching of the areas around the marks in the absence of the mirror was done during the recovery period of some hours that preceded a test. I would note that in experiments with my colleagues Ann Kitchen and Linda Brent, along the same lines, which will be described below, we waited for 22 hours before reintroduction of the mirror. We found as Gallup did, that on reintroducing the mirror to the animals cage, the number of responses directed at the mark dramatically increased—more than 25-fold. The chimpanzee then either inspected its fingers or smelled them. If the reflection were interpreted by the chimpanzee as being another animal, the chimp might have reached towards the mirror and touched the red spot of the reflection. However, its highly co-ordinated motor action of fingering its own red daubed head *guided by the reflection* would seem decisive.

The striking salience is that you cannot examine visually otherwise inaccessible portions of your body with the aid of a reflection unless you know who you are— that is, the animal is aware of itself.

Using this explicit operational criterion of the concept, it would appear that chimps and orangutans have this ability but the data with gorillas are equivocal, notwithstanding the suggestive data on Koko the gorilla, which is in the care of Dr Francine Patterson of California. Macaque and rhesus monkeys, cynamologous monkeys, and gibbons have been negative. A study by Dr Hauser and colleagues (1995) at Harvard used the highly visible and typical head feature of the cotton topped tamarin monkey. They dyed it with a coloured hair dye. This resulted in self-directed behaviour suggesting *on this criterion*, that self-directed behaviour occurred in primates lower than the great apes. Gallup told me that he and Povinelli have not been able to replicate the findings in marmosets.

However, underlying the great complexity of analysis of consciousness, it can be noted that self-awareness has for many years been assessed solely in terms of presence or absence. However, there is no a priori reason to expect self-awareness to be a discrete capacity that an organism either has or does not have, or to expect that one self-aware organism possesses the same level of self-awareness as another. In human children, for instance, the sense of self develops gradually, and manifestations of self-identity vary qualitatively with age. The body image is constructed gradually by trial and error. It is also likely of non-human primates that any self-awareness they possess will vary quantitatively.

Distorting mirrors and chimpanzees

As a further insight on this issue, I wish to describe another experiment on chimpanzees carried out at Southwest Foundation for Biomedical Research in San Antonio, Texas, where Ann Kitchen, Linda Brent, and I (1996) exposed six subjects serially to a convex mirror, a concave mirror, and finally a triptych mirror. In this way the mirrors on successive days confronted the animal with an image of a distorted, very fat short chimpanzee, a very tall thin chimpanzee, or three chimpanzees at the same time. They all had previous mirror experience, including the red mark test. What happened was clear-cut and easily validated from the videotape record.

All subjects exhibited mirror-guided *self-referenced* behaviours, as observed during standard mirror exposure, when they had their first exposure to each of the three types of distorting mirrors. The time that elapsed before the first mirror-guided self-referenced behaviour was recorded. It was less during first exposure to the distorting mirrors than during first exposure to the regular mirror in eight of the 18 first exposures.

On exposure to the distorting mirrors, the subjects displayed little of the social behaviours (e.g. head bobbing, play invitations, begging gestures, and sexual presentations) commonly reported in chimpanzees on first exposure to mirrors; a clear indication that the subjects did not mistake the images for another chimpanzee. In all subjects, exposure to both the distorting or the multiplying mirrors, induced mirror-guided self-referenced behaviours. What happened was that the chimp rocked from side to side and peered at the image intently. The exact contemporaneity of its volitional movement of rocking with the movement of the mirror image allowed quick evaluation of the source of the mirror image. The chimpanzees then largely lost interest, further evidence that they had solved the problem. That is, when confronted with the distorted image *they deliberately swayed from side to side and stared at the reflection doing likewise.* Presumptively, though the reflected image was grossly distorted and presumably unrecognizable relative to any chimpanzee they had seen, it moved with them as they willed themselves to move, and they recognized its movements as their own.

These observations can be interpreted as an indication of self-recognition in all subjects on exposure to all the different distorting mirrors.

Mitchell has described self-aware beings as those with an 'implicitly present mental representation of the organism itself'. It follows that such an animal on exposure to a mirror, will compare the image it is confronted with to its mental self-representation in order to assess correctly the source of the mirrored image. The study I described tested the ability of the subjects to recognize an image that is very different from any mental representation of itself, or any other chimpanzee it may have seen for that matter. *The demonstration of self-recognition in a distorting mirror implies that the subject can abstract.* That is, for self-recognition to occur on exposure to a distorting mirror, the subject must not only be using some other cue or cues, but it must also be able to rationalize and put aside the distortions and validate the image by other means, namely, contingency movement. The chimpanzee appears to be able to use more than one operation to decide 'its me'.

Dolphins

A most interesting advance of knowledge in this area of mirror self-recognition has come from the study of two bottle-nosed dolphins at the New York Aquarium by Diana Reiss and Lori Marino (2001). The dolphins had a plexiglass mirror placed in their pool. They did not show social behaviours in their pool indicative of reaction to a conspecific. The dolphins were marked on different parts of the body that would not be visible to the animal without the aid of a mirror. The marks were about 6 cm and triangular or circular. The position used was such (e.g. under side of the body or behind flippers) that the dolphin would need to orientate its body so as to view the mark. Initially, faked control marking was done at the site to be marked, giving the tactile sensation without any mark being made. Sham marking did not cause any investigation at the reflective surface or any pattern of behaviour that could be interpreted as self-directed. When marked the dolphins spent much more time at the mirror, positioned themselves so as to expose the marked portion of the body to the mirror, and produced orienting or repetitive body movements so that the marked area was visible to the animal in the reflective surface. When marked, the dolphins moved much more rapidly to the mirror, and exposed the marked area for examination. The experiment also involved what were termed, late sham markings, the circumstance being that the animals were sham marked subsequent to the experience of actually being marked. After some experience of being marked the dolphins then showed much more use of the mirror to investigate the touched area of the body, and after finding no mark abandoned any further self-directed behaviour.

Overall, the authors proposed the results showed the dolphins used the mirror to investigate parts of their body that were marked. The areas were otherwise invisible, and in one instance, when the dolphin was marked on the tongue, it immediately swam to the plexiglass mirror and engaged in a mouth opening and closing sequence not exhibited hitherto. Like chimpanzees, they did not maintain a continuous orientation to the mark during a test session, which suggests habituation and loss of interest. Unlike chimpanzees, dolphins did not pay attention to marks on their companions. This was proposed to be attributable to the fact that unlike chimpanzees, they do not groom one another.

Marten and Psarakos (1995) used comparison of real-time self viewed television to try to eliminate social behaviour as a factor in what dolphins did with the mirror. They engaged in elaborate open-mouthed behaviours on self view, but just watched when the material was played back to them. When marked they presented the marked areas to the self view television and turned to do so. The authors felt that the results suggested self-examination.

Anderson (1995) of Strasbourg discussing the data in the field remarks that it is interesting that the dolphins presented with a mirror, or live televised image, self-performed an act so specific as protruding a fish held in the mouth, and then retracting it while watching the self-image. He notes however, that the published studies did not address control experiments in so far as how much twisting was exhibited by marked dolphins in the absence of the mirror. He also reflects that if marked dolphins were to intersperse acts of inspection of the marks with acts of swimming against an object or substrate to try and rub off the mark, their behaviour would more deeply correspond to observed self-recognition in apes where the marked area was touched with an extremity able to do this.

The data raises the issue that mirror self-recognition may not be an element of cerebral organization emergent solely in the great apes, but may reflect the substantial degree of development of the brain in the dolphin. These animals have a high degree of encephalization and cognitive ability. Dolphins have highly developed memory, can reproduce a complex motor sequence (a trick) as a result of observation, as distinct from being taught. This suggests some cognition of their own body image. They show complex social behaviour.

Dolphins diverged from the primate line about 65–70 million years ago, and their brain is different with regard to cortical cellular architecture and organization. Reis and Marino suggest cognitive convergence despite different neuroanatomy and evolutionary history.

Body image and animals

A natural circumstance can underline the complexities of operational analysis of a biological concept. It may not be a controlled experiment, but it is no less real. Thus, turning to the matter of intention as highlighted earlier, we can ask if animals lower in the scale than apes have some rudimentary sense of self? Suppose a monkey with its hand, or another animal such as a cat or dog with its forelimb, strikes an object with that forelimb in the course of an intentional act, and the result is severe pain. This may be associated with sound of striking, and occur within a field of its vision and the result is pain *contemporaneous with its intention*. Would it be aware that its own limb was the source of pain, and, at this level, be aware of that part of itself and thus itself? Or is the situation with the animal similar to that in the human with a particular type of brain lesion, where the patient may be unaware that the paralysed left side of the body is his or her own?

To elaborate this latter point—the following description of this condition of anosognosia in humans, and its remarkable implications, is derived from Antonio Damasio in his book *Descartes' Error* (1994). Deriving from the Greek '*nosos*', meaning disease and '*gnosis*', meaning knowledge, the word means inability to acknowledge disease in oneself. A patient who is entirely paralysed on the left side of the body by a stroke on the right side of the brain and is unable to move that left side, stand, or walk, may respond to the question as to how he or she is, with the answer 'fine'. The patient may be visually aware of the inability to move the left arm and note that 'it does not seem to do much by itself'. Patients with the right side of the body paralysed because of a stroke on the left side of the brain are fully cognizant of their sad predicament. Anosognosia is a phenomenon caused by *right-sided brain damage* of a particular type. It involves also a lack of emotional disturbance in the face of their overall situation. They are indifferent to the fact that a major stroke, which has done this, may herald further problems and they will never be the same.

The remarkable phenomenon of anosognosia appears to be caused by damage to a select group of regions of the somatosensory cortex on the right side involving the anterior of the parietal lobe (Fig. 2.1). The somatosensory system is responsible for both the external senses of touch, temperature, pain, and the internal sense of joint position, state of viscera and also pain. The areas involved comprise the areas that receive sensory inflow from the body on the posterior border of the central sulcus of the cortex of the parietal lobe (S_1), and also the secondary sensory areas (S_2) on the upper wall of the lateral sulcus, mainly behind the primary sensory cortex (Fig. 10.4). The other major component of the group is the insula, which is also buried in the lateral sulcus (Fig. 10.4). The damage involves also the fibre pathways or the white matter. It disrupts connections between these areas cited above, which normally receive signals from throughout the body, and have connections with the thalamus, basal ganglia, and the motor and prefrontal cortex. Damasio (1994) suggests the cross-talk between these areas underpins the integrated map of the current body state. His theory is that the map is skewed to the right hemisphere

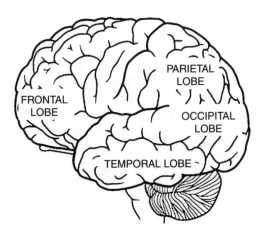

Figure 2.1 The lobes of the lateral surface of the brain.

because of the functional need to have one final controller and this is why the consequences of right-sided lesions are starkly different from those on the left. He sees the region as a co-ordinated dynamic map. It is not contiguous but is an interaction and co-ordination of signals in separate maps. The signals from both sides of the body meet comprehensively there. The left hemisphere representations reflecting the right side of the body are probably partial and not an integrated system.

This structural damage revealing a dismemberment of integration and loss of knowledge that part of the body is part of oneself could perhaps give a hint that at earlier stages of evolution there may be no integrated sense of self. An animal may not recognize that the source of its awareness of pain is a specific part of itself. However, anybody who has playfully teased a cat or dog with small pinches or such-like, and responded to its swift counter manoeuvres would not be too sure about this. Nor would anyone who has watched puppies playing and nipping one another without inflicting damage, be sure that some self-referenced inhibition of strength of bite does not exist. Bite too hard and get bitten back ferociously with real pain.

The issue can perhaps be put more directly as it bears on intention concerning a part of the body.

Explicitly, a situation has been described to me by my colleague Dr Michael McKinley, who has experience of farms in the Australian Alps. Foxes sometimes get their paws and lower legs caught in a jawed trap used for rabbits. The poor animals may frantically go round the anchor point in circles dragging the chain. However, unable to escape in this way, they have been known to gnaw through the lower leg and escape, leaving their paw in the trap. Is the animal aware it is held completely by its paw in the trap jaws, and it has an *intention* to get free? Gnawing through its own skin, muscle, and bone to set itself free is a *purposive* act, and very probably extremely painful. There would seem much more to it than the classical behaviourist black box of stimulus and response, the latter being in the category of reward or punishment. At least it seems a plausible viewpoint that the animal has enough 'body image' sense to see the paw is part of 'itself' that is held, and its intention is to get free. Even if the pain and stress caused massive endorphin release (the brain's natural opiates) in the brain, it seems legitimate to countenance that the animal is aware that part of itself is held. In that sense it is self-aware, and has a plan. The plan is to sever that part of itself that is holding it captive despite the pain—'Wherefore, if thy hand or foot offend thee cut them off and cast them from thee'. (*Matthew 18: 8*).

My friend, Don Watson drew my attention to this passage, and we agree, it is unlikely the brain of the fox embraced the remainder of the text, 'That it is better to spend life as a cripple than to spend eternity intact in hell.'

Donald Griffin has extensively covered comparable issues in his book *Animal Minds* (1992). He notes that an animal capable of perceptual consciousness must often be aware that one of its companions is eating or is fleeing. That is, it would be aware of the actions, and who is performing it. A perceptively conscious animal could scarcely be unaware of its own actions such as eating or running away. If we deny all reflective consciousness (i.e. self-awareness) to such an animal, we suggest its mental experiences entail a large 'perceptual black hole' as far as it, itself, is concerned. This, he suggests, throws into doubt the strong tendency of many scientists to hold that self-awareness is a unique human capacity.

Chapter 3

What some distinguished scientists have proposed on the nature of consciousness: John Searle, Homer Smith, Vernon Mountcastle, and Roger Sperry

I wish now to recount individually the views of some distinguished scientists on the biology of consciousness. The viewpoints are disparate in some ways. However, the overview emergent will outweigh any disjointed sense arising from my sequentially recording the ideas. Thus, as said earlier, the essence of views of neuroscientists and some philosophers that emerges unambiguously over the last century is that mind is what the brain does. Dualism is out. Sir John Eccles, the Australian neuroscientist and Nobel Laureate, is an exception to this. I have discussed with him his rather unusual belief, unusual at least in the scientific world, in the book *The Pinnacle of Life—consciousness and self-awareness in humans and animals* (1995); some detail is given at the end of this chapter.

John Searle

The philosopher, John Searle (1997), thinks it is not difficult to give a common-sense definition of consciousness. This is distinct from an analytical one, which would unveil the underlying essence of the experience. His common-sense definition of the term states

> consciousness refers to those states of sentience and awareness that typically begin when we awake from a dreamless sleep and continue until we go to sleep again, or fall into a coma or die or otherwise become unconscious. Dreams are a form of consciousness, though, of course, quite different from full waking state. Consciousness so defined switches off and on.

Searle gives a lucid outline of the materialist viewpoint in a paper on the 'Problem of consciousness'. He says that, above all, consciousness is a biological phenomenon. It is part of ordinary biological history along with digestion, growth, and meiosis. However, it has features other biological processes do not.

The most important is subjectivity—the sense that each person's consciousness is private to the person. He is explicit that brain processes cause conscious processes, but the consciousness they cause is not some extra substance or entity. It is just a higher level feature of the whole system. But it is a profound problem as to how. Understanding may require a revolution in biology. *Inter alia*, Searle also underlines the fact that our experiences are characteristically structured in a way that goes beyond the structure of the actual stimulus, a profound discovery of the Gestalt psychologists. It has been pointed out, for example by Kandel and colleagues (1991), that Kant's emphasis on preknowledge influenced the emergence of Gestalt psychology, which holds that *aspects of perception reflect an inborn capacity of the brain to order simple sensations in a characteristic way.* Thus our perceptions are not simple records of the world around us. The organized whole that is perceived is more than the sum of its parts. The perceptions are constructed internally, at least in part, according to innate rules and constraints imposed by the capabilities of the nervous system. Perception is not atomistic but holistic—an active and creative process that involves more than just information provided by the retina. You don't see what you're looking at—you look at what you're seeing. The German psychologists, Max Wertheimer, Kurt Koffha and Wolfgang Kohli, who founded the Gestalt school were the first to emphasize this. Crick (1994) has given some excellent visual examples in his book and most readers will, for example, be familiar with the vase that transmutes upon staring into two profiles facing one another (Fig. 3.1).

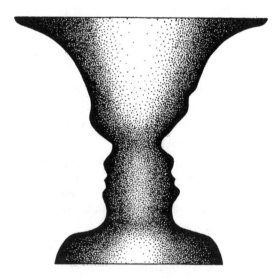

Figure 3.1 A perception change. First it is a vase and then two upturned faces are seen. (Drawn by Mariella McKinley.)

Searle (1985) has also, as Edelman (1992) emphasizes, opposed the idea that any purely computational specification provides sufficient conditions for thought or intentional states. His argument applies to higher order consciousness as occurs in humans. It is that computer programs are defined strictly by their formal *syntactical* structure ('Orderly or systematic arrangements of parts or elements' (*Oxford Dictionary*). However, syntax is insufficient for *semantics*, and in contrast, human minds are characterized by having semantic contents. Semantic contents involve meanings, and a syntax does not in itself deal with meanings. Thus, Searle maintains that in as much as consciousness is identified in humans with a type of intentionality that is inexorably accompanied by subjective experience, by definition no organism can have intentional states if it lacks subjective experience. Computers lack such experience.

Homer Smith

Homer Smith sets out a different slant in a lecture on 'The biology of consciousness' (1959). Homer Smith is honoured for his original discoveries on kidney function. In his lecture he states that the German physiologist Carl Ludwig in 1842 made a major step for the antivitalists. He explained a complicated physiological process like the formation of urine by reference to the same laws as operate in the domain of inorganic nature. Vitalism embraced the idea that the phenomena of life are attributable to a 'sensitive soul' that works directly on chemical processes, an immortal, immaterial principle coming from afar, and at death returning from whence it came.

Smith gives a ringing tribute to Descartes' contribution to science. He defines Descartes' mechanism as designating, in effect, the belief that all activities of the living organism are ultimately to be explained in terms of its component molecular parts. Descartes' statement in the *Traite de Homme* was that of the body as a machine naturally proceeding from the mere arrangement of its organs. It was unnecessary to conceive any other vegetative or sensitive soul embodied in the full description he gave. This was said by T.H. Huxley (1898a) to be in the spirit of the most advanced physiology of Huxley's day. It merely required translation into modern language. Homer Smith (1959) said—'By the opening of the 20th century *the whole of biology had been transferred into what Sir Michael Foster of Cambridge University in 1885 termed "molecular physiology" which meant Cartesian mechanisms at the molecular level.'*

Descartes left animals as curiously contrived machines with no consciousness or feeling. As man's material body is an unfeeling, unthinking machine like the body of any animal, Descartes coupled the mind to the body through the pineal gland. Here, in the pineal gland, mind met matter.

Smith suggests retrospectively he can understand why Descartes left the rational soul in man, since man was so obviously a rational creature, manifesting, in Smith's eyes, modes of behaviour that seemed far removed from any similarities to be observed in animals.

It was two centuries later before the uniqueness of behaviour of humans would suffer serious challenge, indeed, in many aspects terminal challenge. This was as a result of a general theory of biological evolution—i.e. by Charles Darwin.

There is some debate on the influences determining Descartes position in making humans different. Homer Smith (1959) says in a footnote, which I will repeat in full.

> As Descartes 'Le Monde', which reaffirmed the Copernican theory, was about to go to press in 1633, the author learned of Galileo's condemnation by the Inquisition. So he withheld the work. In this and other respects it is recognized that he compromised before the threat of the *odium theologicum*, but whether he is fairly subject to criticism for this self-interest can be debated.

Giordano Bruno had been burned in Rome in 1600 (when Descartes was 4 years old) for rejecting the particularistic propositions of the church (the legend of creation, the Trinity, miracles, etc.) and for incorporating the Copernican doctrine into his pantheism. In 1619 Lucilio Vanini had been burned at Toulouse, and in 1620 Fautauier of Montpellier had been burned at Paris on the charge of atheism. Descartes had no irresistible impulse to martyrdom. He learned that Galileo, now nearly 70 years old, whose essays from 1585 on through the Sidereus Nucius (1610) and Dialogo del due Massini Sistemi del mondo (1632) had stirred the admiration of the learned world, had been cited to Rome by the Inquisition on 1 October 1632. Galileo had been forced to go there on 13 February 1633, to be examined under menace of torture. So Descartes set Le Monde aside, but with the hope that at some later date the authorities would be more favourably inclined toward its publication. As it was, his friends among the Jesuits called him an atheist (for purporting to prove the existence of God) and the Protestants of Holland declared him to be both a Jesuit and an atheist, and he was impelled to seek sanctuary under the Prince of Orange. Le Monde remained to be published (1701) long after his death (1650) because in 1663 his works were placed on the Index. There is, however, no reason to think that fear of the *odium theologicum* played any part in shaping his dualistic philosophy of man.

T.H. Huxley (1898a) says that Descartes saw the discoveries of Galileo meant that the remotest parts of the universe were governed by physical laws, and the discovery by Harvey of the circulation of the blood meant the same laws presided over our own body. Physical science challenged not only philosophy and the

Church, *but also common ignorance which passes as common sense*. The assertion of the motion of the earth was a defiance to all three. Huxley says physical science threw down the glove by the hand of Galileo. The immediate results of the combat were not pleasant. The champion of science, old, worn, and on his knees before the Cardinal Inquisitor signing his name to what he knew to be a lie. Two hundred years later, physical science sits crowned as one of the legitimate rulers of thought. As Huxley put it 'The Cardinals—well the Cardinals are at the Ecumenical Council, still at their old business of trying to stop the movement of the world.'

Smith (1959) thinks that in proposing animals are unconscious automata, Descartes made a great mistake, in that he might otherwise have speeded up development of biological science and philosophy by at least a century. As a result of his position there came later a body of opinion that stated the other extreme. That is, both humans and animals alike become conscious automata.

Homer Smith looks upon Thomas Henry Huxley as one of the greatest scientists of a great century. Huxley (1898b) stated apropos evolution 'The doctrine of continuity is too well established for it to be permissible to me to suppose that any complex natural phenomenon comes into existence suddenly and without being preceded by simpler modifications; and very strong arguments would be needed to prove that such complex phenomena as those of consciousness first made their appearance in man.'

However, Homer Smith (1959) finds elements of Huxley's position on consciousness difficult to understand.

Assuming, however, that 'molecular changes in the brain are the causes of all states of consciousness', Huxley doubted if there was any evidence that these states of consciousness might conversely cause those molecular changes in the brain that give rise to muscular motion. He thought the consciousness of brutes would appear related to their body simply as a *collateral* product of its working, and to be as completely without any power of modifying that working much as the steam whistle which accompanies the work of a locomotive engine is without influence on its machinery (1898b).

As a diversion here of possible interest, Tolstoy used the same locomotive analogy in his discussion of the forces that determine the movement of humanity. 'A locomotive is moving' Tolstoy writes, 'and someone asks what moves it—a peasant says it's the devil, another says, because the wheels go round, and a third says, the cause lies in the smoke which the wind carries away.' The man that says the movement of the wheels is the cause refutes himself, in that once he goes on to explain why the wheels go round he may reach the ultimate cause of movement, which is the pressure of steam in the boiler. Tolstoy says that the only conception which can explain 'the movement of whole peoples is that some force commensurate with the movement is involved.' He notes that various historians take forces that are not commensurate with the whole movement of peoples. Some see it as a force inherent in heroes, some as a force from several other factors akin to the movement of the wheels, and others 'as intellectual influence like the smoke being blown away.'

Huxley felt that mental conditions are simply the symbols in consciousness of the changes that take place automatically in the organism. Further, that the feeling we call will is not the cause of a voluntary act. It is the symbol of that state of the brain that is the immediate cause of the act. These days, of course, Huxley would have the advantage of neuroimaging, and the fact that volitional imagination of motor intention can cause direct changes in physiological functions within the brain, just as imagination of visual or auditory experience does. Interestingly as well as involvement of the motor cortex area, imagination of movements in a tennis game activated middle and caudal parts of the cerebellum bilaterally.

For Homer Smith (1959), the word *consciousness* meant a very specialized activity of the nervous system without any transcendental implications. As observed subjectively in oneself, consciousness is not an 'all or none' phenomenon. Clearly it varies in intensity, complexity, and pattern in the waking state. It waxes and wanes, and ceases to exist. It utterly disappears in dreamless sleep. From a neurophysiological viewpoint, its presence or absence in experimental animals and humans is generally characterized by certain typical features of the electroencephalogram. Homer Smith felt it had been progressively developed in the animal kingdom *in special relation to the mobility of the organism, to the necessities of going from here to there.* He reflects that all animals are dependent on either plants or other animals for food. The evolution of the animal kingdom has presented a pageant of predator and prey—eat or be eaten! This was the issue of evolution of consciousness.

The mobile predatory habit required the successful animal to solve the Cartesian problem of the moving bodies but in four dimensions. Space and accurate timing was a *sine qua non*. Accurate timing required the integration of events in the recent past with those of the present moment, allowing extrapolation into the future. Smith proposed that given the short duration of individual neural events in the periphery, the problems of going from here to there could only be solved by fusion of rapid neural events into a continuous or persistent image in which elapsed time appears as a dimension. He sees this neurophysiological fusion as the essence of consciousness. *Thus the unique feature of consciousness is its time binding quality, its persistence beyond milliseconds into seconds, or even minutes.* He thinks that there is no requirement for awareness of the environment or self in the individual organism until it develops to the point where it possesses the physical freedom to go from here to there. It needs the neuromuscular system necessary to take advantage of that physical freedom. Hence, Smith says, one need not look for consciousness in the entire non-motorized plant kingdom. Evolution occasionally leaves useless things in its wake, but it does not create them *de novo* (Smith, 1959).

Homer Smith's intuition of the need to go from here to there in pursuit of food brings to mind a later statement by J.Z. Young, 'No animal can live without food. Let us follow the corollary of this. Food is the most important factor in the evolution of the brain and the behaviour the brain dictates' (Young, 1986).

Vernon Mountcastle

Vernon Mountcastle of the Johns Hopkins Medical School, is a great pioneer of cellular studies of brain systems. He discovered that single nerve cells of the primary somatosensory brain cortex respond to specific kinds of touch. These cell types make up vertical columns over the 2 mm depth from cortical surface to the white matter below it. Each column is an integrating unit. David Hubel and Torsten Weisel (1997) found similar vertical columns in the occipital pole of the brain cortex (the visual area). They responded to lines of a particular orientation. Their discovery provided an entirely new view of the anatomical organization of the cerebral cortex. Subsequently, investigations of vision have revealed that some 30 or more areas of cortex subserve the visual process. Information arising initially in the V1 area at the back of the occipital area is analysed in two parallel processing streams. The dorsal or top stream is concerned with where objects are located in space, and how to reach them. It extends from V1 to the parietal cortex. The lower or ventral stream goes forward to the inferior temporal cortex. It is concerned with analysing the visual form, and colour of objects. Perception of an object in space engages a diverse group of neural areas that process different aspects of the visual information. As Semir Zeki of University College, London, puts it, 'The visual percept does not reside in any given visual area, even if that area is critical for certain features of that visual image. Rather, it is the result of on-going activity in several re-entrantly connected visual areas.' (Zeki, 1993).

This general background serves to introduce Mountcastle's general view of the problem of consciousness and that of describing it. He proposes that it will eventually be defined in terms of neural mechanisms, as organisms without nervous systems do not display observable attributes of it. Consciousness appears in animals along with the development of a complex nervous system.

He thinks it is difficult to draw any line separating those animals that are from those that are not. It is better to regard species as distributed along a continuum of increasing degree and complexity of consciousness. He says: 'The presence of the conscious control of action may, as an operational definition, be assumed when an organism displays the capacity for choice of action, the ability to set one goal aside in favour of another, the power to withhold action or reaction.' (Mountcastle, 1980).

Mountcastle suggests a high order of consciousness is involved in anticipatory planning for action, in changing action once begun in the face of what is happening, and in preparing options to deal with images of what might happen. This is a property of brains termed intelligence.

He says publicly observable behaviour in humans and animals suggesting presence of consciousness includes:

1. Attention, and ability to shift it selectively.

2. Manipulation of abstract ideas, particularly using symbols or words—characteristically in humans. However, there is evidence of elaborate communication between individual animals of many species. (Donald Griffin would see the symbolic dances of honeybees as an exemplar of symbolic communication.)

3. Capacity for expectancy, and in the case of animals in the wild by tool use, by organization of troops for hunting and by posting of sentinels.

Parenthetically, it could be noted here that the criterion of the emergence of mankind used by Kenneth Oakley of the British Museum was tool making. It involved the making of an object for an imagined eventuality. In this sense, it is akin to Aristotle's definition of the artist.

In relation to Mountcastle's idea of distribution along a continuum, the tool making by chimpanzees (stripping a branch of its leaves in order to fish in a termite mound for ants), would be paralleled by the propensity of the otter to bring up a stone from the sea bed under one arm and say, a clam under the other. The otter will float with the stone on its chest, and bang the shellfish against the stone to split it open. When the shellfish is eaten the otter then discards the shell but may retain the stone and dive again. It returns with a new shell to hit against the same stone. This implies some anticipation of the use to which the stone is to be put.

The view of W.H. Thorpe (1966) of Cambridge University was that the most precise example of anticipatory hunting behaviour is that recorded by Jane Goodall of the chimpanzee troop organizing themselves so that one or more of their number attracted the attention of a colobus monkey. Thereupon another chimpanzee crept up behind and leapt on the monkey, which was then seized by all and torn to pieces and eaten. Expectancy is dealt with in Chapter 4 with regard to behaviour of fish.

4. Self-awareness is indicated by social and familial behaviour of animals, by their organized play and their imitative behaviour. Also copying of novel acts or utterances is indicative.

To me it is cogent in relation to Mountcastle's emphasis on this behaviour that imitation of the novel action of a conspecific implies an awareness by the initiator of its own body image in order to volitionally move elements of it in appropriate sequence in order to mirror the actions of another. There are striking examples of dolphins blowing bubbles and imitating humans, such as divers using aqua lungs, and who are cleaning the glass walls of the dolphin aquarium. Dolphins imitate elaborate tricks that other dolphins have been taught without having had any tuition themselves.

5. Aesthetic and ethical values can be considered as emergent lower in the phylogenetic tree than Homo sapiens. The behaviour of bower birds, and the reciprocal grooming of chimpanzees are possible cases in point.

Mountcastle also discusses the variable intensity, as it were, of consciousness in a given individual. It varies from alertness to drowsiness, and, in general, reduction of sensory inflow results in a reduction of consciousness, though, in complex nervous systems, imagery may supersede this effect. Consciousness presupposes memory with continuous storage of information about internal and external events. This is a record against which anticipatory action is planned.

The overall level of consciousness depends, in general, on the excitability of the brain, and this is determined by the reticular activating system (RAS). The ascending RAS extends from the medulla and midbrain to the thalamus (Figs 3.2 and 11.2). It lies parallel to and receives collateral input from the great afferent (sensory) systems travelling from the periphery of the body to the thalamus. It is driven thus indiscriminately though the inflow may be organized topographically—i.e. inflow from different parts of the body going to different parts of the RAS. It tunes the ongoing levels of excitability of the cells of the cerebral cortex, the basal ganglia, and other large grey structures of the forebrain. It sets the stage for action, and its function has been termed generalized. Destruction of it causes loss of consciousness.

Mountcastle (1980) goes on to say that the so-called specific afferent systems (that is, the big nerve trunks carrying touch and other sensations to the brain) that operate in parallel to the RAS are precisely organized for transfer of such information. This is in contrast to the general arousing and alerting function of the RAS. Without the sensory inflow the animal is blind, deaf, or without

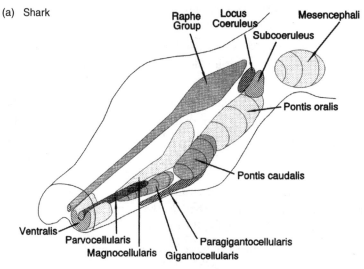

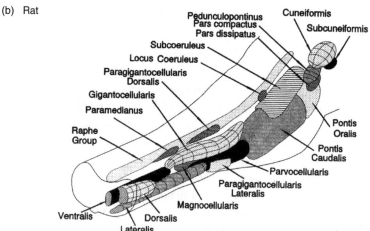

Figure 3.2 (a) The main cellular groups of the reticular formation of a shark. (b) The main cell groups of the reticular formation of a rat. As the authors point out, the structure is well conserved in all jawed vertebrates, and the main components can be recognized. From Ann Butler and William Hodos *Comparative Vertebrate Anatomy*, Wiley-Liss, New York (Publishers), 1996. (With kind permission).

sensory feeling. Without the latter it cannot be aroused from a sleep-like state. Almost all areas of the cortex receive projection fibres of the two types. *Jean Pierre Changeux, (1985), of the Pasteur Institute and College de France, has likened the RAS to the console of an organ, which can be played and direct attention to particular areas of the cortex.* In a neuroimaging study using positron emission tomography (PET) by Kinamura, Per Roland and colleagues (1996), at the Karolinska Institute in Stockholm, the activation of the midbrain reticular regions together with intrathalamic nuclear groups was clearly shown when attention was aroused in conscious humans (Fig. 10.5).

The comparative anatomists Ann Butler and William Hodos have given a detailed description of organization of the RAS in animals as varied as lamprey, shark, lizard, and rat (Butler and Hodos, 1996) (Fig. 3.2). Their analysis, they suggest, designates the reticular formation as one of the systems that has been conserved from the primitive vertebrate brain right up the phylogenetic tree to humans. The main components of the system are recognizable in all jawed vertebrates, and the chemical pathways involving noradrenaline, serotonin, dopamine, and GABA-ergic neurotransmitters are also conserved (i.e. present in all). A reasonable suggestion emerging from these comparative data is that this arousal system, which activates the rostral brain (i.e. the forward part of the brain called the telencephalon), may be ancient, and function comparably in lower animals.

Roger Sperry and the split brain

Before dealing with our main question of the beginning of consciousness with progressive ascent of the phylogenetic tree, it would be remiss not to consider one of the most remarkable of all investigations of human consciousness. That is, the surgical splitting of the brain in the midline, which results in the individual having two minds. It gives fascinating insight into brain function, and also has droll and direct implications in relation to aspects of theological thought. The brain is split down the middle into right and left halves by division of the corpus callosum, which is the great commissure joining them. It carries about 200 million fibres connecting the two sides. This was done in humans to prevent spread of severe epileptic seizures. Some minor commissures are divided also—anterior and hippocampal. The experiments were carried out by Roger Sperry of the California Institute of Technology with his colleagues Michael Gazzaniga, Joseph Bogen, Philip Vogel and Evan and Dahlia Zaidel and others. Initially Sperry (1974) had shown that division of the corpus callosum in monkeys and cats allowed experiments in which one side of the brain could be taught one response and the other side another, and even conflicting response to the same situation. When the operation has been done on humans he said that everything indicated that the surgery has left the people with two separate minds. That is with two separate spheres of consciousness. What is experienced in the right hemisphere is quite outside the realm of awareness of the left hemisphere in relation to perception, cognition, volition, learning, and memory. The left hemisphere in the right-handed person is dominant or major. It is talkative and conversant, whereas the other, the right hemisphere, is mute and can express itself through non-verbal reactions. As Sperry puts it, the surgery gives mental duplicity but not 'double talk'.

The functional divide between the two hemispheres is counteracted by many unifying factors, which tend to have the two hemispheres doing the same thing most of the day. However, when experiments deliberately induce different activities in the right and left, it becomes evident that each hemi-sphere is oblivious to the understanding of the other. For example, if the patient was blindfolded and a familiar object put into the left hand, e.g. pen-cil, cigarette, or coin, the left hand connected to the right (mute) hemisphere knows what the object is. However, it cannot express the knowledge in speech or writing (which is controlled by the left hemisphere). It can manip-ulate the object and show how it is supposed to be used and retrieve it with the left hand from a group of objects by touch. However, the other hemi-sphere will say, if asked, that it does not know what it is, or it will guess. If the right hand is allowed to cross over and touch the object it can immedi-ately say what it is.

The same division is seen in tests involving vision. The right half of the field of vision projects to the left talking hemisphere whereas the left hand side of vision projects to the right (Fig. 3.3). In these patients visual stimuli flashed to the right side of a central visual fixation point and thus transmitted to the left talking hemisphere are easily described and reported correctly. However, material flashed to the left field and transmitted to the right hemisphere is lost on the talking hemisphere. The right mute hemisphere can pick out an object with the left hand if the picture is flashed, or the word for it is flashed in the left visual field. If an object were flashed, it could pick out the word for it. Further to this, it is possible to divide photographs in half longitudinally, thus joining the faces of two different people. This makes what is termed a chimera. Thus with central gaze the left brain sees one face, the right the other. If the patient is required to match the photograph to what is seen, the right mute hemisphere dominated. If the patient were asked to name the image, the left hemisphere dominated. The right mute hemisphere was found to be ineffec-tive with arithmetic. But it could draw an object like a cube with the left hand whereas the left hemisphere was no good at it even though it had the right hand to do it with. A most interesting finding was that if the divided photo-graphs flashed were of beautiful or ugly people, the right mute hemisphere was very proficient on delineating aesthetics, whereas the left hemisphere could not tell beauty from beast.

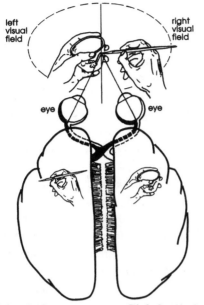

Left hemisphere

- faculty of speech
- right-handed skills
  such as writing
- verbal memory

- superior
  comprehension
- calculations

Right hemisphere

- left-handed manipulation
- memory for shapes

- mute: limited
  comprehension
  of language
- superior
  comprehension
  of topography, faces

Figure 3.3 A diagram of a split brain (corpus callosum divided) showing that information coming to the retina from the right visual field feeds by the optic nerve into the left hemisphere, whereas the stimuli in the left visual field feeds into the right hemisphere. The faculties that are dominant or advantaged in the left or right hemisphere of a right-handed person are shown. (Drawn after C. Trevarthen.)

Sperry (1974) has also reported emotional feelings generated by the right mute hemisphere, such as a smile when a task is completed with the left hand, or frowning at incorrect verbal response, or inept action by the right hand, when only the minor mute hemisphere knows the correct action.

During the early stages after operation there was evidence of each hemisphere having a will of its own, and the two did get into conflict with one another. A particular instance Sperry described was with one patient dressing and trying to pull on his trousers. The left hand might work against the right and try and pull them down on the other side. There was an instance when the sinister left hand sometimes tried to push the patient's wife away aggressively at the same time as the hemisphere of the right hand was trying to get her to come and help with a task.

Notwithstanding this evidence of dysfunction, important emphasis on the coherence of behaviour of split-brain persons is given by Dahlia Zaidel (1994). She notes, *inter alia*, that many subcortical channels could and seemingly do achieve coherence between two sides of the brain. Indeed, she says, in daily life the patients appear to behave as if there were no evolutionary purpose to this major neuronal connection between the hemispheres. Some functions such as speech and language comprehension appear unimpaired. Further, previously learned functions that require interaction between the two sides such as riding a bike, swimming, or playing the piano, appear unchanged over the years. Changes in personality are not evident, and intentional behaviour is not restricted to the dominant speaking hemisphere. That is, in daily life, either right or left hand may reach out to pick something up. They appear to have a unity of central consciousness characterized by awareness over short periods of time (termed the horizontal dimension of unity by John Searle), and also simultaneous awareness of a number of perceptions as part of consciousness (termed the vertical unity by John Searle).

However, after disconnection of the hemispheres new bimanual movements are learned only after exceptional difficulty. In considering how the daily habitual learned behaviours are controlled, Zaidel considers that such behaviours may be integrated in subcortical structures, and raises the interesting possibility of unified cerebellar control being involved with other subcortical structures.

Insight on this issue came from experiments by Pashler Michael Gazzaniga and colleagues (1994). The psychological refractory period is overt when two stimuli are presented in succession to a subject and independent responses to each are required. If the interval between the first and second stimulus is decreased, it increases the time for the second response to begin because the second response has to wait until the selection of the first response has been completed. This is seen in normal individuals even if the two tasks are easy or involve different hemispheres. Gazzaniga and colleagues compared normal individuals with four split-brain subjects. They posed the question that if the interference of one task with the other involved corticocortical connections between the two hemispheres, as, for example, might occur in responding to stimuli to the two differing visual fields each relaying to its specific hemisphere, then this form of dual task interference should be eliminated in those who had had the commissure severed. If the contrary were found, it would give evidence that subcortical structures play a critical role in co-ordination and sequencing of cognitive processes. All four of the split-brain patients showed dual task interference very similar to that found in normal individuals. Thus subcortical structures play a part in co-ordinating multiple streams of sensorimotor performance, and their role may be critical for the remarkable intactness of bilaterally coordinated behaviours in the everyday life of split-brain patients.

However, 'split-brain' patients do suffer evident impairments. Recent memory suffers dramatically after surgery. Topographical (that is memory of locality or place) is particularly poor, and such patients have great difficulty in locating a parked car or items around the house. They lose interest in reading newspapers or watching TV, probably because of loss of integrating memory. Emotional sexual arousal achieved by feeding visual information into one hemisphere (e.g. the right) is experienced by the left, but without any capacity to interpret verbally what has happened.

There are accounts in the literature going back to 1940 of 'diajonistic dyspraxia', designating conflict between hands as a result of damage to the corpus callosum. A.J Akelaitis (1945) coined the term meaning division with fight or struggle. The French neurologists M. Poncet, E. Barbeau, and S. Joubert (2001), describe cases and also material in the literature. These involve struggles between the left and the right hand, whether it be putting on clothing, but with the left hand trying to pull the item off, opening a door with the right hand and the left hand seeking to close it, and so on. They also describe more complex behaviours where the patient carries out an action, e.g. putting on shoes and tying the laces, and then unties them, takes the laces out of the shoes and throws them away. Also, a patient may set the table for dinner, and then when it is done takes all the plates, glasses, and cutlery, and put them away in cupboards and drawers. Often it can involve paralysis of the ability to decide between alternatives when, for example, shopping.A proposed generalization from the data ranging from surgical division of the corpus callosum to partial damage to it from cerebrovascular lesion, which includes the data of Tanaka and colleagues (1990) from Japan, suggests that the abnormal behaviours limited to the hands were the result of lesions to the ventral posterior corpus callosum. Pathways connecting the two superior parietal lobes traverse there. The lobes are thought to be involved in selection of movement. However, lesions also involving the anterior corpus callosum, which connects the two front lobes give rise to disorganized executive behaviour—stopping or no normal sequential behaviour with a meal or the morning toilet, and starting a procedure and becoming, in essence, paralysed.

An interesting new insight on self-recognition has come from study of split-brain patients. A group at Harvard, Keenan *et al.* (2001), have shown neural organization of the right hemisphere seems to be preferentially involved in the process of self-awareness. They studied a group of patients undergoing the Wada test, which involves the inactivation (anaesthetization) of one cerebral hemisphere. This is done to gain information regarding which cerebral hemisphere is dominant for language. This is in relation to the treatment of epilepsy. The test involves administration of the anaesthetic amobarbital into the carotid artery on one side for a brief period. Five right-handed patients (the left hemisphere is dominant for language) were shown pictures of faces made by morphing (melding) the picture of a famous person with the patient's own face. Patients were instructed to remember the pictures presented and different pictures were shown. After recovery from anaesthesia, they had to choose which face had been shown—i.e. their own or the famous person. That is, the choice was between the two faces that had made the morph—a photograph of their own face or, the photo of the face of the famous person. Neither face, only the morph, had been presented during anaesthesia of the one or the other hemisphere.

Following anaesthesia of the left hemisphere, during which the right hemisphere would still have been awake, all patients (five of five) selected the 'self' face as the one that had been presented. However, with anaesthesia of the right hemisphere leaving the left awake, four of the five selected the famous face. The results suggested that the anterior right hemisphere may be critically involved in detecting the 'self' face. The authors suggest these most interesting results may be generally congruent with the clinical data of anosognosia and asomatopagnosia involving neglect and lack of recognition of one's own extremities *after stroke on the right side of the brain*. The authors suggest that the fact of self-recognition in a mirror by humans and the great apes, but not monkeys, may be indicative that the neural circuits subserving this capacity are only recently evolved.

Sir John Eccles, an Australian Nobel Laureate for his contributions to knowledge of synaptic transmission, wrote extensively on the mind—body hypothesis. He was unusual among neuroscientists in accepting the earlier doctrines of a transcendental mind separate from the brain. He had a theory that the bundling of the dendrites or processes of neurons in the lower layers of the brain cortex as they extend up the surface of the cortex gave a functional entity called a dendron. His theory of mind—brain interaction resided in the linkage of units that he called 'psychons' to these dendrites. A mental intention, which is an immaterial phenomenon, would act through a psychon. The world of mental events has an existence as autonomous as the world of matter-energy itself.

In 1992, I had the pleasure of discussing the mind—body problem bearing on Descartes onwards with Sir John in Switzerland. Eccles had been the convenor and editor of 'Brain and Conscious Experience', a study week of the Pontifical Academy of Science in 1964.

At this conference held at the Vatican, the Pope had addressed the assembled eminent group, and it was after returning from the meeting that Sperry remarked to his colleague Michael Gazzaniga (1985) that the Pope had said, in essence, that the scientists could have the brain, and the Church would have the mind.

Discussion with Sir John Eccles on dualism

In the discussion with Sir John (see *The Pinnacle of Life*, 1993, 1994, 1995) our consideration of the brain–mind issue inevitably led to Sperry's investigations.

I reproduce below the verbatim record of the discussion because it would seem a rather fundamental theological issue emerges.

DD: Concerning the right mute hemisphere, I had referred to the fact that the patients sometimes behave as if there were two people there—the sinister left hand that used to proceed to undo buttons in opposition to the right—as if there were, in effect, as you were saying, two people.

JE: Yes, that's what I'm saying too. I agree with that, but there isn't . . . the right hemisphere with this mute person. The conscious self is not, I think, a proper self in the human sense of the word, because it's not a person. It doesn't make decisions in the light of foresight, imagination, value systems and so on. This is what is missing in the performances that you get out of the right hemisphere.

DD: With respect of aesthetics, it is capable, certainly, of initiating actions in the face of the knowledge it has—I mean of objects, and so on. In a sense it's a separate stream of consciousness . . .

JE: Yes, but it doesn't have a proper value system in grading its actions, as far as one has been able to see from all these experiments. It is, as it were, a kind of automaton in a way, and not making subtle judgements. In the considerations, it doesn't worry about the future and the consequences of its actions. Things like that. This is what is missing. So what I would say . . .

DD: Are we sure that capacity is actually located? I mean, obviously, the articulation of it is in the left hemisphere in the right-handed person, but are we actually sure that it's in the left hemisphere that such judgements are embedded, as it were?

JE: Well, Sperry is trying to say with his very advanced techniques that there is evidence that the right hemisphere does worry about the future because he puts it through all kinds of testing for whether it believes in an insurance policy and things like that, but I have not been convinced by these at all. I do not think that it knows what that insurance policy is. It has no good understanding of the subtleties of language. So by and large . . .

DD: It's not good at mathematics, is it?

JE: No. Good at geometry, but not in arithmetic. But there is a position that I think I accept. Namely, that there are two conscious beings, you might say there, separated by the section, but not two human persons with selves in the ordinary sense of the word. Responsible, you might say . . . Responsible, highly motivated human selves. The other one, it is just a performer but not a self.

DD: *Does that mean you would in effect put the soul in the left hemisphere in the right-handed person?*

JE: *Yes. Well, but not, no, no, but when the corpus callosum is cut.* When it's not cut, both hemispheres are working much more together. We do not understand or allow for this nearly enough. You cut the corpus callosum, and then you think you have got two separate hemispheres, one and the other. In real life, with two or three hundred million fibres firing at one another from almost all parts of the cerebral cortex, the cortex is one—an entity . . . And this cutting of the corpus callosum is, shall we say, very rough treatment of this, and not one that's going to give you any subtle judgements about the functions of the left and right hemispheres.

DD: You agreed that it shows, in a way, two separate conscious processes, as you've said. And in a way, wouldn't that—coming back to the first point that I made—wouldn't that in effect indicate that consciousness is an outcome of neural tissue in action, and you can have these two relatively separate neural tissues—two relatively separate, and with different capacities, streams of consciousness?

JE: Of course, but then that is still misunderstanding the brain-mind problem in dualist interactionism, because what one is saying in dualist interactionism is that they are so closely locked together, the mental and the neural, interacting in a most subtle way, and with any of our tricks we can't separate them. But not that they're independent, in a sense that the initiative of action comes from the mental in all of our decision-making, in all of our ordinary human actions. It's the mental that leads the neural, but this is a very intense interaction going on. And it's not just going one way. It's backwards and forwards like that. That, I think, has not come into consideration in criticising dualism.

I have noted in retrospective comment on this that, whereas Sir John initially said 'yes' to the soul being in the left talking motor hemisphere of the right-handed person with cut corpus callosum, he immediately abdicated the position though he had rather conceded several times that there were two conscious beings with the split-brain patient. The conjecture that arises theologically comes from the fact that with people living with split brains, eventually it may occur that someone will have a stroke that destroys the left interpretive and talking cortex. Would such a person be thereupon deemed to be without a soul, though all the appreciation of beauty and aesthetics sometimes equated to highest human sense of value would be intact and functioning in the right hemisphere? The right hemisphere as Sperry points out can make judgements of colour—qualia. Or, if as Sir John did, one retreats from the initial position that the soul is in the talking, mathematically enabled hemisphere, does it follow, as it is agreed that both hemispheres are conscious, that there are correspondingly now two souls in the patient? Is it a case of split soul?

Furthermore, in relation to Sir John's argument that the right hemisphere of the right-handed person is not a real self in the ordinary sense of the word but just a performer, there is now information that was not available to Sir John at that time. I refer to the Harvard experiments on the morphs, recounted above, which put self-awareness in the right hemisphere—not the left—a conclusion also emergent from the data on anosognosia or hemi-neglect.

There is, also perhaps an interesting and somewhat amusing judicial conjecture. Whereas split-brain patients integrate reasonably well, emotion may be generated by either hemisphere and it is conceivable that visual information of a nature to generate high emotion could go predominantly or wholly to one hemisphere. A scenario of great improbability would be if a split-brain patient given to some suspicion walked along a passage and applied his or her left eye to a keyhole at an angle such that the right visual field saw their partner having sex with someone else. He or she, so enraged, grabs a revolver sequestrated nearby with the left hand, and rushes in and shoots dead both people on the bed. As the hand controlled by the hemisphere receiving the information could pick up a pistol and shoot, presumably the hemisphere in control of the hand used would be legally responsible. The issue could revolve around whether only the hemisphere that knew about it was guilty and the other innocent. In some countries, happily few, decisions on this could determine which hemisphere should be executed.

These questions, though they have some of the same attraction as the old issues of how many angels can dance on the head of a pin, do perhaps point to the relativity of aspects of moral judgement of behaviour. It might be argued that it is not an instance of diminished responsibility of the hemisphere that was executive as it would be fully cognizant of its intention. The situation is that the other hemisphere knew nothing about it. However, it can be noted to give perspective to this quite implausible scenario, that Dahlia Zaidel (1994) recounts that split-brain people do not appear to react typically to death or divorce with bitterness, sadness, hatred, anger, or violence. They don't speak of revenge or violent acts. They react to situations in a factual way (i.e. that's the way it is), and this may include infidelity. There is no deep insight, but it is not to say they don't experience sadness, infidelity, loss, or anger.

Chapter 4

Consciousness in animals

The idea of a goal is an integral part of the concept of mind, and so is the idea of intention. An organism which can have intentions, I think, is one which can be said to possess a mind... To form a plan and to make a decision—to adopt the plan.

The idea of forming a plan in turn requires the idea of forming an internal model of the world

Christopher Longuet Higgins
(see Kenny 1973)

The peculiar feature which defines intentionality is that it is a property of mental life that refers to entities that are not observable at the time. Intentional thoughts are different from other purposive thoughts where the aim is clearly in view... *it is the state of an individual who is planning or expecting action with reference to some condition of affairs that is not immediately present.* (My emphasis)

J.Z. Young (1986) (Discussing views of Brentano and J.D. Searle)

If we can see purposive behaviour in animals or men, we have provisional grounds for believing that there is within the organism some expectancy of the future which entails or implies a capacity for ideation, an integration of ideas about past and future, and a temporal organization of ideas.

D.O. Hebb (1949)

Take your favorite sensory motor routine in some species and enforce a waiting period of a few seconds between the sensory input and the execution of an action. If the subject can't perform the task with the delay, it was probably mediated by a zombie agent. If the organisms performance is only marginally affected by the delay, then the input must have been stored in some sort of intermediate short term buffer, implying some measure of consciousness. If the subject can be successfully distracted during this interval by a suitable salient stimulus (e.g. flashing lights) it would reinforce the conclusion that attention was involved in actively maintaining information during the delay period.

Dogs, probably like all mammals easily pass this test. Think of hiding a bone well out of sight and teaching the dog to sit still until you tell her to 'go fetch the bone'.

Christof Koch (2004; a Turing test for consciousness)

Intentional behaviour at different levels of the phylogenetic tree

These four quotations above represent a primary basis for attribution of mental processes to animals. The idea of consciousness as an appropriate challenge for direct physiological analysis was regarded for a good part of the twentieth century as an arena for the misled or philosophically inclined rather than for the disciplined experimental scientist. The strict behaviourist approach as exemplified by Watson (1913) and Skinner (1971) had a big influence in this regard. The brain was a 'black box'. What we knew was only revealed by the behaviour induced by stimuli. In the field of animal behaviour it acted to avoid any anthropomorphic explanations of what was observed. This was because explanation by analogy with the human experience could involve the assumption of conscious awareness and often self-generated intention, which has an essential subjective element. Skinner's (1971) behaviourism was most radical in so far as he relegated questions concerning inner mechanisms, whether involving neural mechanism or mental states to the improper. He wrote— 'The emotions are excellent examples of the fictional causes to which we commonly attribute behaviour.'

Happily for the advance of knowledge, the emphasis has changed over the last few decades. There has been an explosion of analysis of consciousness with many books by eminent biologists and physicists, as well as emergence of journals devoted to the subject. The scene has changed dramatically. It has been said by Yngve Zotterman, a pioneering Swedish neuroscientist, that 'in science the excitement lies in hunting the big game'. There is great enthusiasm in the present pursuit of new insights into consciousness both by experiment and debate.

Dramatic advances in analysis of consciousness involved, *inter alia*, the discovery by use of positron emission tomography (PET), and functional nuclear magnetic resonance imaging (fNMRI), that it was possible to record local discrete increases or decreases of blood flow in specific local regions of the brain during explicit changes in the conscious state in humans. Blood flow changes are believed to reflect corresponding local increases or dampening of neural activity. In appropriate experimental circumstances, these could be related to a sequence of changes of the stream of consciousness occurring at the same time. This has ignited optimism that real advances in understanding the neurophysiological basis of consciousness may be possible—albeit tempered by recognition of the seemingly incredible complexity of the problem. Crick (1994) points out that a main problem is determining among the protean areas of the brain that light up or inhibit in a given situation, which ones are related to consciousness and which ones are not. We will allude to important aspects of the complexity of this problem later. However, it has led some to the belief that the problem may never be solved. Denis Horgan, a senior writer for the Scientific American, in a book *The Undiscovered Mind* (1999), has suggested that 'When it comes to the human brain there may be no unifying insight that transforms chaos into order'.

There are discernable directions of transition from the extreme behaviourist era to the current climate. It is now fairly common for scientists to consider the responses of an animal in terms of conscious processes that may cause them. They will use terms that imply such processes.

The aim was to have a discipline of analysis with explicit terminology. However, it was recognized that behaviour was exceedingly diverse. The simple attribution of behaviour to instinct had been discredited. This was because it had been used as an explanatory force obscuring the need for further analysis. However, it came to the forefront again with the recognition that internal bodily states (hormone or chemical changes) had a major role in generating behaviour. Also they might determine whether or not external stimuli had an effect or not.

The instincts or genetically preprogrammed behaviour patterns were central to the behavioural analyses of the Nobel Laureates Tinbergen and Lorenz. They used terms such as 'action specific energy' to characterize the build up of excitability in the brain directed to a particular end. This central excitability set in motion genetically programmed motor activity. This happened when the stimulus predestined to be apt, and thus relevant to the genetic determined organization, turned up. This specific sensory stimulus was called the innate releasing mechanism, which set the behaviour in motion.

In parallel to the ethologists, Curt Richter, of Johns Hopkins University, the great pioneer of psychobiology, showed how need states in the animal could cause the development of appetites and intake behaviour precisely apt to the animal's need. The needs were contrived by deprivation of intake of substances obligatory for survival, or by surgical removal of an endocrine gland, which caused loss of minerals from the body, or by hormone administration. The fact of specific apt choice in the absence of any prior experience of the situation spoke for the genetic programming of the behaviour. Experiments at the Howard Florey Institute in Melbourne on sheep have determined some of the chemical mechanisms in the brain underlying specific appetite behaviour for essential minerals. Parallel contribution to basic knowledge has come from, *inter alia*, Epstein, Stricker, Johnston, and Schulkin in the USA, Fitzsimons in the UK, and Nicolaides in France. Richter also showed other forms of behaviour such as nest building can occur with changes in the internal hormonal status of the organism.

An essay directed to the formal analysis of behaviour entitled 'Motivation', by Eliot Stellar (1960) of the University of Pennsylvania, reflects the directions of advance away from the position of the behaviourists. Donald Griffin had called behaviourism 'the mindless science'. Much of Stellar's analysis concerns self-regulatory behaviour such as hunger and thirst. He emphasizes that operational definition of the concepts used for laboratory analysis of behaviour is possible. Such operationally defined concepts in motivation include drive, goal-directed behaviour, and satiation. Directed drive is measured by strength of consummatory behaviour as, for example, that in the face of obstruction. An example would be whether or not an animal would cross an electrified grid to get to the goal. Drive can be produced by deprivation, hormonal changes, and other fluctuations in the internal environment. The greater the drive the greater the activity, the greater the consummatory response, the greater the energy expended and the work done. However, increasing drive beyond a certain point may reduce motivated behaviour because of physical impairment of the animal.

Whereas the psychobiologists have made great advances within this framework, it is notable that the general slant of the viewpoint involved in their analysis is to the intentional side of behaviour. *Inter alia*, drive is defined in the *Oxford Dictionary* as an organized effort to achieve a particular purpose. Whereas it is implicit that the motivation or drive arises for a particular reason, the emphasis is much more upon the action than it is on the imperious sensation that gives rise to the intention and how that imperious and specific sensation is generated in the brain. The genesis of this imperious specific sensation is as much a hard-wired event, as the concomitant intention or motivation.

The major leader in bringing consciousness in animals to the forefront of experimental enquiry and discussion has been Donald Griffin of Rockefeller and Harvard Universities. Early on, he made outstanding studies of echolocation in bats. His several books, including *Animal Minds* (1992), cover work by many scientists bearing on a basis for attribution of conscious processes to animals.

In considering the first emergence of primary consciousness, the argument can be made that a certain number of neurons, a mass of sufficient size, is necessary to sustain a process of such complexity. This conjecture of itself highlights some striking anomalies if there were a predisposition to relate neural mass to the level of, or complexity of, conscious processes. Table 4.1 derived from one published by Dr George L. Gabor Miklos (1998) of the Neuroscience Institute of La Jolla, California, reflects this. The comparison of the number of neurons of the honey bee (850 000) with the number in the octopus (150 000 000) is salutory. It will serve to introduce a discussion on the behaviour of the octopus and *Sepia*—most interesting and, in some ways, versatile invertebrates.

Table 4.1 Approximate gene and neuron numbers in the brains[a] or entire nervous systems[b] of organisms in different evolutionary lineages

Organism	Genes	Neurons
Worm	16 000	302[b]
Fly	12 000	250 000[a]
Miniature wasp	NA	5000[a]
Honey bee	NA	850 000[a]
Marine snail	NA	20 000[b]
Octopus	NA	520 million[b]
Puffer fish	70 000	NA
Miniature salamander	NA	300 000[a]
Laboratory mouse	70 000	40 million[a]
Human being	70 000	85 000 million[a]
Whale and elephant	70 000	200 000[a]
Tobacco plant	43 000	0

NA, not available. Reprinted from Miklos, G.L.G. The evolution and modification of brains and sensory systems. *Daedalus (Journal of the American Academy of Arts and Sciences)*, **127**: 197–216, 1998.

Invertebrates

J.Z. Young (1964, 1986) made pioneering studies on the octopus. Young proposed that the supraoesophageal brain centres (see Fig. 4.1) of the cephalopods are large and allow study of effect of removal of large parts of the nervous system on behaviour and learning. These centres probably evolved relatively recently—possibly in the last 10 million years. As shown in Table 4.1, the octopus has about 520 million neurons, with 150 million in a richly inter-connected brain involving centres such as the optic lobes, and the correlation centres occupying the dorsal area of the brain. The other 370 million neurons are organized in ganglia at the base of its arms.

The correlation centres termed the verticalis complex allow interaction between impulses from different inflow sources. They send tracts to motor centres and the optic lobes (Fig. 4.1). These vertical lobes are electrically silent. That is, electrical stimulation does not cause movement.

The main action patterns of the octopus are generated in the basal lobes, which are in the lower part of the supraesophageal mass. These areas are concerned with the action patterns of attack and retreat. Electrical stimulation of these areas causes the animal to rise up, turn its head, and walk towards the side stimulated. If the lobes are lesioned or removed an animal may walk or swim in circles, and sometimes do it for many hours.

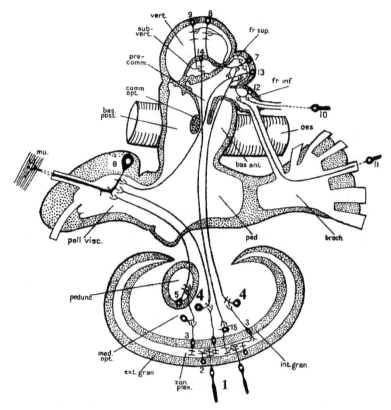

Figure 4.1 A diagram of the octopus brain showing the verticalis (vert) and frontal lobes (fr), which are dorsal (above) the oesophagus (oes). These lobes may be analogous to the limbic system in mammals. The basal posterior (bas post) and basal anterior (bas ant) lobes generate the attack and retreat behaviour of the octopus. Below (ventral to) the oesophagus is the optic lobe with the retinal cells (1) feeding to it. It is the target part of the brain and as shown, neuronal outflow (4) from it leads to motor cell controlling muscles, but also to the verticalis and frontal lobes, which assess reward and punishment. (From F.K. Sanders and J.Z. Young. *Journal of Neurophysiology*, 3: 501–525, 1940. With kind permission of the American Physiological Society.)

The optic lobes dealing with vision and visual memory have more neurons than the verticalis and the superior frontal part of the octopus brain, which appears to be involved in the relevance of signals indicative of reward. J.Z. Young points out this is a most important function for an exploratory self-teaching homeostat (a self-regulator of its physicochemical status). He thinks functionally these two lobes may be analogous to the limbic system in mammals. Octopuses need the right amount of exploratory drive to probe their environment. They give credence to reward or punishment. As he sees octopus behaviour, they are encouraged by success but not to the point of rash risks. They are cautioned by pain but not to the extent of being depressed to inaction. An exploratory homeostat needs to acquire this optimum balance. These lobes appear to subserve the ability to learn this basis of existence. Furthermore, they have the capacity to bridge the time gap between a signal to the distance receptor (the eye), the process of pursuit and capture, and then eating of the prey giving rise to the sense of reward involved.

In relation to an octopus being an explorer, Young says that it must attack unfamiliar objects or it will not learn anything. This may involve motivation or intention governed by a need. However, little is known about hunger in octopuses. However, after a large meal there is a much reduced tendency to attack. But it must learn to attack objects that have yielded food and avoid those that don't, or hurt it. In the latter case it must again retain the information from the distance receptor until the result of action arrives. It can then accordingly change the probability of response. That is, learn the consequences of particular actions. There is evidence that the octopus can maintain a balance between the tendencies to do or not to do a particular thing.

Studies by Maldonado (1963), of University College, London, have shown an octopus fresh from the sea when first shown a crab in its tank will leave its home and then attack only after a significant time. This time is greatly reduced after several experiences, and so also is the time of movement between the home and the prey. It was interesting if the light was turned out at various stages of the attack. It was found the attack could be finished in complete darkness, indicating that some programme or plan existed in the brain. Pain signals such as associating an electric shock with a crab or with a rectangle, which previously signalled crab, result in no further attacks for a period—sometimes of several days. After the shock it withdraws and swims to its home. There may be an elaborate withdrawal pattern involving change of colour. Eventually, it may put its arms over its head, particularly if further shocked. The possibility is that large fibre tracts reach or pass the subvertical lobes and carry the pain signal.

Young with his colleague K.F. Sanders published a paper on the related cephalopod *Sepia*, a decapod, which was entitled 'Learning and other functions of the higher nervous centres of *Sepia*' (Sanders and Young, 1940). After surgical removal of the verticalis lobe there was no apparent change in the *Sepia*. It could move around normally and steer, and was not blind. In terms of eating, it showed a normal reaction to a prawn. It approached it, seized it, and ate it like a normal *Sepia* would.

However, a characteristic of the *Sepia* is to hunt. This situation was contrived experimentally by having a prawn attached to a piece of cotton. The prawn could be drawn around an upturned bucket in a tank and then around an enamel plate which was behind the bucket to reach an end-point at C (Fig. 4.2).

Sanders and Young (1940) point out that in the experiment the *Sepia* needs to follow its prey twice (i.e. around two corners) after the latter has passed out

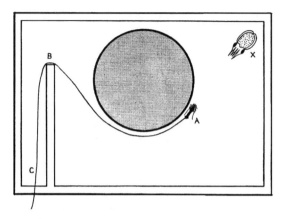

Figure 4.2 Figure of the experimental design of a tank used by Sanders and Young to show capacity of *Sepia* (the cuttlefish) (X) to hunt when its prey (a shrimp on a cotton) (A) passes out of its sight, and goes around a corner (B) to a point (C). The *Sepia* will pursue the shrimp—sometimes after an interval of 2 minutes before beginning to do so. (From F.K. Sanders and J.Z. Young. *Journal of Neurophysiology*, 3: 501–525, 1940. With kind permission of the American Physiological Society.)

of sight. It tests the capacity of the animal to make a response to a situation where no directly stimulating object is in its visual field. To put it another way, it tests whether the animal is able to retain the association of a particular locality with its food object when the food is no longer present there, and to use this association for its hunting. The experimental set-up mimicked to an extent the circumstances in nature. A *Sepia* would need to follow a prawn that had disappeared out of sight. It will go round the corners to eventually seize it at C. Sometimes the whole reaction is rapid and complete within a minute or two. On other occasions the animal *waits for as much as 2 minutes before gradually turning the corners to pursue the prawn*. The authors also raise the question of a cephalopod being able to pursue an object by a devious route as being indicative of 'intelligence'. However, they do not explicitly record whether this happened with *Sepia*.

After removal of the verticalis complex, the *Sepia* was unable to hunt but could catch a prawn only if it remained in its field of vision. Sanders and Young (1940) consider the potentiality of self-re-exciting circuitry between the optic lobes and the verticalis in subserving this behaviour. However, the issue of 'the corner around which the prawn had disappeared' at least 1–2 minutes before does provoke a question. That is, of the *Sepia* retaining some image in its brain to direct its behaviour consonant with the Turing test proposed by Koch and Crick. It is suggestive that the behaviour would reflect an attention and intention with some dim consciousness. However, a distraction was not included in the study to see if the putative attention might be disrupted. However, the capacity is demonstrably served by some 150 000 000 neurons in aggregate, and explicitly lost with removal of the lobe. So the question does arise. Dr Edward Bullock (1982), the distinguished comparative physiologist of San Diego, and E. Basar have shown the electro-encephalogram of the octopus brain indicates that many neurons are functionally synchronized to generate low frequency field potentials, which are comparable with those of the vertebrate brain. It is also noteworthy that in the description of the behaviour, the *Sepia* were described by Young as hungry, or 'when hunger drive operated' as when the attack occurred. After feeding they were described as 'satiated'. In his book *Model of the Brain*, Young (1964) notes that there must be receptors that indicate the 'needs' of the animal, e.g. for food, and he says further—'After a large meal the octopuses showed a reduced tendency to attack'. It is not known whether this period of satiation is related to the fullness of the crop, nor by what pathway the relevant impulses pass to the brain.'

The filling of the crop could be analogous to the distension of the stomach and occurrence of satiation in higher vertebrates. However, a question arises as to whether hunger is subserved also by any component of the circulating fluids acting upon sensors in the body (interoceptors) giving an action on the brain. Bullock and colleagues have data suggestive of an internal sensor reacting to blood glutamate levels. Rhanor Gillette (1991) of Illinois has been a leader in the study of the invertebrate nervous system. He has stated that work on cephalopods has been motivated by the complexity of their intelligence and lured by the presence of great neural complexity in a line evolved independent of that leading to vertebrates.

A further fascinating instance of octopus behaviour under experimental conditions has been reported by Graziano Fiorito and Pietro Scotto (1992) of the Zoological Station of Naples. Individual octopuses learned to discriminate between two balls of similar size but different in colour (red or white). Attacking the correct coloured ball resulted in a small piece of fish as a reward. Attacking the wrong ball caused the animal to be punished by an electric shock. The first group of octopuses, called 'demonstrators', learned which ball to attack, and training was considered completed when the animals made no mistakes in five trials. A trial lasted about 40 seconds and the intertrial interval was 5 minutes. Then untrained octopuses, called 'observers', were housed in an adjacent tank with full visibility through glass. They were allowed to watch four trials in which the 'demonstrators' attacked the right ball even though the 'demonstrators' were *not* rewarded for making the correct response. Video recordings showed the 'observer' octopuses increased attention and followed the 'demonstrators' with their eyes during the four trials. They spent more time outside their homes. They displayed other behaviours seen in *Octopuses vulgaris* when in the presence of a member of the same species. Thereupon the 'observer' octopuses were given five trials of the procedure. They made the right choice of ball as was done by the demonstrators, even though no reward was given the 'observers' for the right choice. The outcome is that an octopus can learn a task by observing for a short period of time the behaviour of a conspecific. As a commentator remarked, 'Octopus see and octopus can do!' Furthermore, the learning was stable, as it persisted with trials carried out over five consecutive days. Observation is therefore a powerful mechanism of learning in this species.

In Fiorito and Scotto's (1992) view, such copying of a model by an invertebrate, appears related to the cognitive abilities of the learning system of vertebrates. One interesting question that comes to mind with this fascinating data is whether the same learning would occur if the demonstrators were not conspecifics? Thus, does the exclusively visual appraisal carry any implication of cognition by the octopuses that this was done by one of themselves? After all, presumably they have to know something of this sort in terms of configuration in order to mate? Tinbergen's experiments suggest it is colour pattern as well as type of movement which allows an octopus to recognize the opposite sex.

Correspondence in *Science* subsequently raised some objection to the interpretation of the experiment. Suboski, Muir, and Hall (1993) noted that the octopuses had learned which stimulus to respond to, not how to respond to it. This is a typical act that can be acquired through social learning. Biederman and Davey (1993) proposed that, a control experiment was required to separate the role of the stimuli from that of the 'demonstrator'. Fiorito and Scotto (1992) state that points raised, such as that it was rapid imitation involved, are semantic in so far as imitation is considered a form of observational learning.

The question of what in invertebrate behaviour is representative of more than mere mindless circuitry, and what might be solely innate chain reflex behaviour has been studied by J.L. Gould and C.G. Gould (1986), of Princeton University. They recount that the female of a species of digger wasp may maintain simultaneously several burrows containing developing offspring. In the morning the female visits each of the concealed tunnels and checks on the offspring. As a result of this inspection she knows which burrows still contain eggs that don't require food, which are occupied by young larvae that will need two or three caterpillars to eat, those that have older larvae, which will need many more caterpillars, and those containing newly pupated offspring that need to be sealed off to allow development to be completed. On the basis of the visit to these five or 10 underground nurseries the wasp knows how much prey to capture and where to take it. On the face of it, the behaviour looks thoughtful and demanding. If the residents of the various burrows are switched the next night (i.e. before the morning inspection) the wasp has no difficulty in stocking each nursery appropriately the next morning. However, if the changes of inhabitants are made after the morning inspection, the wasp is mindless of the fact the burrow now has an egg instead of larvae. It will spend the day stocking it with caterpillars as if it still contained older larvae. This is even though the wasp may touch the eggs many times during the day. Young larvae may be sealed off because previously the burrow had contained a pupa. The wasp shows no hint of insight—it is oblivious. It is programmed by the initial stimulus.

On the other hand, these workers experimented on honey bees. They found that if they used an artificial food source, and systematically moved it further and further away from the hive on each trial, some of the trained foragers would, as it were, 'catch on', and anticipate subsequent moves and wait for the feeder at the presumptive new location. It could be taken as an impressive intellectual feat. It is not easy to imagine anything in the behaviour of natural flowers that might have caused evolution to programme bees to anticipate regular changes of distance.

The Goulds' recount another intriguing experiment, whereby they trained foragers beside a lake (Gould and Gould, 1986). They tricked them into the dance characteristic of bees, which indicated to the recruit bees that a food source was in the middle of the lake. Recruits refused to search for these food sources even when they put food in a boat in the lake. They wondered whether the bees had some phobia to water. However, when they increased the distance and put the food on the opposite shore of the lake, the recruits responded to the dance and turned up in great numbers there. On the face of it, the possibility considered was that the bees 'knew' how wide the lake was, and distinguished between sources supposedly in the lake and on the opposite shore. The experimenters were unable to account for this behaviour on the basis of associative learning, or trial and error. The simplest account seemed to be in the postulate that the recruits had mental maps of the surroundings. They somehow position on these the spots indicated by the dances.

In an overview the Goulds' make a cogent observation. Does the apparent ability of the bees to make and use maps provide convincing evidence of active intelligence? And if so, why are bees so completely mindless in other contexts? They say that if they were designing an animal they would 'hard wire' as much of the behaviour as feasible. If there is a best way of doing something it would seem pointless to force an animal into a time-consuming mistake prone and the potentially fatal path of trial and error. However, if explicit programming will not serve the situation, it seems better to direct the organism to fall back on 'thinking'. This is particularly so when the solution to the problem can be wired into the system for later use. They add the point that much of human behaviour falls into such a frugal neurological pattern. We work hard to master a problem but eventually the solution becomes a mindless automatic behaviour. For example, difficult problems like learning to type, ride a bicycle, drive a car, tie shoes laces, or knit, seem extremely difficult initially, but, once learned, become quite matter of fact, like walking. In the overview they see a continuum of complexity rather than dramatic difference with the ascent of the phylogenetic tree.

Fish

The structure of the bony fish forebrain is relatively simple because it has no neocortex and limited differentation only. As Overmeir of the University of Minnesota, and Hollis of Mount Holyoke College in the US point out the teleost—the bony fish—cannot be regarded as representing a distinct stage in the development later on of other existing vertebrates (Overmeir and Hollis, 1990). However, they are advanced relative to their Devonian geological era precursors which also gave rise to the separate line culminating in the land animals. There is debate among comparative anatomists about their brain structure. They have no neocortex. Some think the differentiated areas of the fish telencephalon are homologous with limbic structures of the more complex brains of higher vertebrates.

Experimental work has shown that fish show a number of capacities comparable with mammals. Habituation involves reduction of response to a stimulus after repeated presentation or prolonged exposure. It is often considered indicative that features of a stimulus have been processed, assessed as noninformative, and remembered. Thus, habituation is a waning of attention. It has been shown that fish have habituation behaviour. Further, that removal of the telencephalon of the brain impaired that habituation in fish. This is in contrast to Pavlovian conditioning where the circumstance is that a neutral stimulus (CS) precedes in time a strong unconditioned stimulus (US) such as food, and then the CS takes on the property of controlling a behaviour. It is the simplest form of association learning. In fish, the removal of the telencephalon does not effect this association learning.

Furthermore, in fish, the presentation of a pleasant event like food or a sexual partner, or *termination* of a punishing event such as an electric shock can be made contingent upon performance of a particular behaviour—*instrumental conditioning*. With this, the designated behaviour becomes more vigorous. If the reward is kept close in time to the response, removal of the telencephalon does not influence it.

However, in avoidance learning the events are arranged so that a few seconds after the presentation of a brief CS, a US like an electric shock is due to occur. This Pavlovian type pairing will hold unless the animal makes a specific instrumental response. *Thus the animal learns to instrumentally prevent an electric shock*, and after a few trials makes the instrumental response as soon as the CS comes on, and prevents the US (the shock). The action becomes vigorous. Thus, as Overmeir and Hollis (1990) point out, this is a conundrum. The puzzling question is as to how the *omission* of an event can function to reinforce avoidance behaviour. After all, if the animal makes the designated response, nothing happens. *The non-occurrence of an event can be meaningful only if the animal expected the event.* Thus the issue of expectancies—a cognitive construct—presents to behaviour analysts.

Though total removal of the telencephalon had no effect on Pavlovian conditioning, such extirpation of the telencephalon dramatically impaired this instrumental avoidance learning.

Overmeir and Hollis (1990) suggest that instrumental avoidance is dependent on brain mechanisms different from simple Pavlovian conditioned reflexes or simple instrumental learning. *Excision of telencephalon impairs utilization of expectancy for control of acts.* In terms of species characteristic behaviour, excision of the telencephalon causes also a large decrease in aggressive behaviour in stickleback fish, jewel fish, sword tails, and fighting fish.

Argument against or favouring consciousness in fish

The issue of whether some dim awareness could occur in fishes, is disputed by Dr James Rose (2002) of the University of Wyoming. His argument centres on the proposal that fish cannot experience pain. It is accepted that consciousness is necessary to experience pain. He notes that awareness of pain in humans depends on specific regions of the cerebral cortex. Fishes lack these brain regions, and thus, putatively, lack the neural requirements necessary for pain experience. Correspondingly, conscious experience of fear, similar to pain, is a neurological impossibility for fishes. Dr Rose's arguments are directed to countering the contention that fish can experience pain. If they could, aspects of their treatment in sport and commercial fishing are not humane. He says this appears to influence regulation of the use of fishes in research. It is a typical instance of anthropomorphic error.

Rose (2002) says that the proposal of Donald Griffin that consciousness may exist in diverse non-mammalian vertebrates and invertebrates, does not take account of the fact that consciousness depends on neocortical functioning. Thus, the proposal lacks feasibility. The cerebral hemispheres of fish have a more rudimentary structure that differs substantially from the structure of the mammalian cortex. Also, reptiles have a simple three-layered general cortex as distinct from the six-layered mammalian isocortex. He notes that as all forms of human consciousness require neocortical functioning, two conclusions arise. First, that non-mammals cannot have consciousness because they lack the neural requirement. Second, perhaps these lower organisms are able to generate consciousness by a different neurological process. This second option might be regarded as an open question.

The key to Rose's (2002) position is that fish reaction to stimuli and injury that would be painful in the human is a nociception process. That is, nociception, as Patrick Wall, the great English authority on pain put it, is an activity induced in a nociceptor and nociceptive pathways by a noxious stimulus. It is not pain that is a psychological state. Invertebrates, which have no brain, show reactivity to noxious stimuli, *per se*, indicating this reactivity can occur in the absence of awareness of such stimuli. Similarly, with only brainstem and spinal cord alone, animals are capable of fully exhibiting typical pain-like reactions to injurious stimuli. This occurs also in people with extensive cortical damage who are without consciousness, or in infants born without cerebral hemispheres. Rose notes that nociception in the periphery of the body sends impulses via the spinothalamic track to the reticular network processes. Such input generates innate behavioural responses such as withdrawal, facial grimacing in higher mammals, and vocalization.

In sharks, the nociceptive fibres do not have much representation in the inflow to the spinal cord. This is not the case in bony fishes, which have an ascending pathway analogous to mammals.

Rose notes that the fact that morphine can reduce reaction to electric shocks in fish. Its effect is counteracted by naloxone (a morphine antagonist), which suggests that a nociceptor response is occurring in response to the shock. However, in his view, this does not demonstrate the conscious experience of pain. This is because the actions of these compounds are at lower subcortical levels of nociceptor processing. He thinks that if some pain awareness were possible in the brain of fishes, its properties would necessarily be so different as not to be comparable with human-like experience of pain and suffering. Any proposal of pain in fish must have a mechanistically plausible neural basis. His overview being—fish lack the neural organization for anything comparable with that in the mammal.

Rose's dissertation written in 2002 was anteceded among others, by an article in the *New Scientist* in 1992 by Patrick Bateson, the Provost of Kings College, Cambridge, and Professor of Ethology at the University of Cambridge. In 1987 he had been a member of a committee of the Institute of Medical Ethics, which had proposed animals can feel pain. This is if receptors sensitive to noxious stimuli are present in functionally useful positions in the body. Bateson notes that the way humans readily project their emotions and intentions into some animals and not others is a cause for concern. However, few people have much fellow feeling for fish. He suggests that observable signs associated with subjective sense of pain in humans are useful criteria for assessment of pain in other animals. On the other hand, considering animals generally, different species react differently to potentially damaging situations. He says stimuli that make a human run and scream might make other animals such as rats, or cattle, or horses, immobile.

Ann Butler, as mentioned earlier, has written with William Hodos a great scholarly work on comparative neuroanatomy (Butler and Hodos, 2005). Butler has kindly communicated some views to me on the possible capacities of the fish telencephalon. Generally, her view is that behavioural response to a noxious stimulus in fish does not necessarily imply either a conscious experience of the stimulus or an emotional distressing response to it. She would agree that consciousness is a prerequisite to experience of pain and its distressing emotional aspect. She considers the proposal put forward by Rose that the neocortex, particularly its association areas such as prefrontal, anterior cingulate, and posterior parietal, is essential to conscious distressing pain experience in humans, and possibly in other animals. She suggests there are objective neuroanatomical reasons that allow for other possibilities.

Butler (personal communication) examines as one example, the human (mammalian) striate cortex, and form vision. 'Striate cortex in mammals is essential for fine form and colour vision. This region of neocortex is quite well understood in terms of its columnar organization and the laminar localization of processing that occurs within it. In contrast, birds lack neocortex entirely. Their Wulst (a bulge or swelling on the dorsal surface of the cerebral hemispheres that receives visual and sensory projections) is well established as the homologue of mammalian striate cortex. However, most of their fine form and colour vision is carried out by the entopallium, the visual part of the clearly nonlaminated dorsal ventricular ridge. Thus, while the laminar neocortex of area 17 is essential for form vision in mammals, birds have a structure with a markedly different cytoarchitecture that can do form vision very nicely. Again, more than one type of neural substrate can perform a given function. Even farther afield, fish do form vision with their optic tectum. It is much more elaborately laminated and developed than the superior colliculus is in mammals.'

Thus, she says, she cannot agree that as non-mammals lack neocortex, they may not consciously experience a variety of stimuli, including distressing sensations up to pain. Rose has noted that 'neural functions depend on specific neural structures,' and 'the neural processes mediating conscious awareness appear to be highly complex, requiring large, structurally differentiated neocortical regions with great numbers of exactly interconnected neurons.' However, Butler would argue that as rats and birds have form vision (with birds better than rats by far), these criteria are primatocentric and may not be valid for all animals. Highly complex, exactly interconnected pallial regions occur in a variety of animals and may thus be a sufficient neural substrate for some conscious perceptions.

Butler goes on to say that across the range of ray-finned fishes, the range of variation in telencephalic development is huge. Some, such as cladistians (e.g. the reed fishes), have very little cell migration away from the ventricular surface in the pallium, and it is hard to believe that they could have consciousness with that pallium. On the other hand, a number of the teleosts (bony fishes) have a very enlarged and elaborate pallial structure (the dorsal part of the telencephalon that presents cell architecture, which is to some extent cortical and in layered fashion, or is cortical plus nuclear groups).

Butler agrees that we cannot assume that non-mammals have a conscious, 'emotional reactivity and pain experience' similar to that of humans. However, if neural substrates other than neocortex can produce form vision and cognitive representations, they may also allow for the experience of emotional distress. In animals, such as birds, with particularly large forebrains, and particularly large brain–body ratios, this possibility must be strongly considered. In some fishes, particularly those with the large brain–body ratios, one cannot entirely rule out the possibility.

Apropos the basis of Pavlovian conditioning in fish, Stephen Walker (1983), remarks that it is necessary to take into account the possibility that animal behaviour reflecting past experience is doing so by unconscious processes, or even simpler mechanisms, which should be distinguished from interesting forms of internalization of knowledge. To illustrate the point, he considers an animal that withdraws into its shell in response to a vibration. Now, suppose it gets a spaced-out sequence in which each vigorous vibration is preceded by flashing lights. Although the animal does not normally withdraw in response to flashing lights, it is now found that it does. This looks like a Pavlovian conditioned reflex, and it might be postulated the creature had the capacity for associative learning like Pavlov's dogs did. However, Walker suggests that if the neuron from the light detector reached the single synapse in the vibration–withdrawal circuit, the theory could be advanced that conjunction of activity at the end of the light detector neuron with transmission across the synapse due to the vibration had somehow melded the light detector into the circuit. It could then activate the withdrawal neuron itself. There would not be any need to propose that the animal had any independent memory of light–vibration pairing, or was subject to vibration expectancies when exposed to flashing lights.

Reptiles

Gordon Burghardt (1991) of the University of Tennessee has written in a very entertaining and forthright way on the matter of mental phenomena in reptiles. He has given great credit to Donald Griffin, who has led attempts to establish a study of animal minds (cognitive ethology) to break the shackles of the mindless behaviourism. In particular, Burghardt states, for him, the attraction of Griffin's attitude is that he discounts the dogma that large brains are critical for cognitive processes—including thought and awareness. Griffin has considered this in honey bees and other insects. He argues that 'thinking' may make up for the lack of brain tissue sufficient to have all contingencies 'hard wired' genetically. He laments, however, that Griffin and others have ignored reptiles though they are the derivations of ancestral stock from which both mammals and birds arose. He says they should be studied as phylogenetic precursors of complex behaviour. May be it is not necessary to assume these processes began in endotherms (i.e. animals that depend on the internal generation of heat). They could have happened in reptiles, which operate on a slower time scale.

Burghardt (1991) states that it is one thing to assert that conscious awareness is essential to all cognition as defined by psychologists, which includes the simplest kinds of learning, and another to use cognitive functioning as evidence of conscious awareness. From Romanes (Darwin's contemporary and colleague who assigned emotions and intellect to reptiles based perhaps on anthropomorphic grounds) to Griffin, awareness and consciousness are indicated by, but not restricted to, complex behaviour involving choice or decision. In his approach, Burghardt does caution that ethologists jumping into the fray of debate too often have not carefully considered the implications of bandying around common-sense mentalistic terms in relation to animals. This is notwithstanding how obviously valid they seemed to be.

Burghardt has given an extraordinarily interesting description and analysis of death feigning in a hognose snake. He remarks that finding food and shelter may be critical. However, nothing produces an acute crises more threatening to continued existence than a sudden confrontation with a predator.

The snake when approached by a human may coil, puff up its body, expand its neck like a cobra or hiss or blow. After other actions, it may develop an erratic writhing behaviour, defecate, turn over, and finally become quiescent—mouth open, tongue extended and with no evident breathing. It can be carried, poked, and there is no further sign of life. If the human instigator leaves and later returns, the snake will be gone. Darwin recognized this death feigning as a means of escape from predators and thus the operation of natural selection. Such immobility responses have been described in birds and many mammals. Donald Griffin has used the fact of versatile adaptability of behaviour to changing circumstances and challenges as a widely applicable criterion of conscious awareness in animals. Burghardt (1991) proposes this applies to the behaviour of the hognose snake. He notes that this defensive behaviour of the hognose snake is highly variable in its specifics across members of the same litter. Such variability, he proposes is common among the complex responses of animals in which we are most likely to look for mental processing of information. One of the experiments that Burghardt did was particularly provocative. The recovery period from death feigning was recorded in three conditions.

1 In the presence of a person looking directly at the snake from a metre away.

2 With a person in the same position but with eyes averted from a direct gaze at the snake.

3 In a control condition in which the person moved out of sight as soon as the snake became quiescent.

The presence of the human increased the time before recovery, with direct gaze having the largest effect.

A similar result was seen if a mounted stuffed screech owl was suspended on a tripod one metre from the snake. The experiments were done on neonate (recently born) hognose snakes and suggest the animal possess good visual acuity and can use the ability to modify behaviour in a sophisticated way.

Overall, Burgardt (1991) argues that with the death feigning of the hognose snake, the descriptive and the experimental data meet Griffin's characterization of conscious awareness in animals. That is, being associated with cognitive processes involving an adaptive response, variability, and a context specificity. He adds that the reader can decide whether the snake is conscious. But posing the question with a snake rather than a chimp makes the study of animal consiousness less affected by uncritical anthropomorphic biases.

Apart from the work on snakes, studies of learning and other behaviour have been made on turtles. As noted by Alice Powers (1990) of St Johns University, this is a fortunate choice in relation to interest in the evolution of the brain as turtles are the best living representative of the ancient reptiles that gave rise to mammals. In the turtle there is no true neocortex. A six-layered cortex does not exist outside the mammalian brain.

However, individual regions resemble areas of neocortex in receiving visual, somatosensory and auditory projections from the thalamus. There is cholinergic innervation (use of acetylcholine as a transmitter) as is the case in the cortex of mammals. Lesion studies in turtles show that learning is impaired by damage to the forebrain regions that use acetylcholine as a transmitter.

To consider briefly the question of image memory—Stephen Walker (1983) has given an analysis of work on 'image-memory' by Beritoff, who worked in Pavlov's laboratory in St Petersburg, and initially studied conditioned reflexes. The story is that he began to examine more complex situations after he observed a dog react by running downstairs after it saw a piece of meat thrown out of a second floor window. This he followed up by experiments where a dog in a cage was shown a piece of food that was then hidden behind one of several screens, and the dog let out of the cage several minutes later. If it went directly to the food then image memory was attributed to it. The fact that the memory was still there if the dog went to sleep and woke up 30 minutes later argued against pointing being the basis of its correct choice. Furthermore, the fact that after 2 hours it couldn't make the correct choice and operated randomly argued against smell being the cue. Beritoff endeavoured to compare this 'image memory' in different species. The memory was very limited in the case of goldfish. In the case of a large aquarium divided into three sections, they were able to swim back directly into the section in which they had been fed if placed back at the starting point within 10 seconds. Longer than that, they simply swam down the middle. Whereas, on the face of it, 'image memory' appeared to exist, it persisted for a brief time only. However, Culum Brown (2004) has shown Rainbow fish improved escape response towards a novel trawl in their tank with a sequence of experience, and retained the memory when tested 11 months later.

Frogs learned to go to a feeding tray in response to a light. But only after scores of feedings in which a worm was put on the tray 10 seconds after the lamp was turned on. They learned also to swim away from electrodes that delivered painful shocks.

Lizards and turtles, however, showed behavioural evidence for 'image memory' similar in kind to that obtained from dogs. The reptiles were confined to a part of their living quarters, shown a piece of food being hidden within their field of vision, and then released to see if they could retrieve it. They got it right if released within 2 or 3 minutes, but not after longer intervals. In particular, if some obstructions were deliberately placed in the direct path to the food, the animals climbed over it or detoured around it. These results indicated a considerable flexibility of the reptilian behaviour. Considered in the context of the earlier description of the variable performance of the hognose snake recounted by Burghardt (1991), they focus the analysis on Donald Griffin's criteria of consciousness in animals, and also, perhaps Longuet Higgins' focus on intentional behaviour that bespeaks an image in the mind. Beritoff's experiments showed that with lizards and turtles, if they were allowed to partially eat the food, and then removed, they were only able to return to the place if the interval was no greater than 2–3 minutes, which was not the case with birds for example. Baboons were able to make the correct choice if released from their cage up to 30 minutes later.

In baboons, as well as dogs and cats, it was possible to demonstrate memories lasting weeks or months if they were carried into a room and given food in a particular place, and then released at the door of the room weeks or months later.

Sleep–wakefulness cycle

One proposition that can be put forward in terms of comparative study of behaviour is that consciousness will occur in those animals that have a sleep–wakefulness cycle. Indeed, this is to an extent implicit in John Searle's (1997) definition of consciousness detailed at the outset. This idea could be elaborated further to put the crucial emphasis on dreaming during sleep. If this were confined to mammals it would give a line of demarcation between thinking and dreaming vertebrates on the one hand and the lower vertebrates with life dominated by reflex behaviour. Stephen Walker (1983) has raised this issue, but has pointed out that this situation does not hold as far as birds are concerned. They may have a dream life not very different from mammals. It may be that a dichotomy will emerge between warm-blooded vertebrates that dream and cold-blooded ones that do not.

Certainly it is clear that birds are diurnal. Many birds that use perches sleep while standing up. The grip on the perch is contrived by a particular muscle arrangement that operates when the main musculature is relaxed. It has been established in some bird species that up to 50% of the day is taken up with sleeping and about 10% of this involves rapid eye movement (REM) sleep. This is true in pigeons and two species of birds of prey that have been tested. The electroencephalogram (EEG) data indicate the brain rhythms character-istic of dreaming are not a mammalian preserve.

At the extreme, Ralph Greenspan and Bruno van Swinderen and colleagues (2000, 2002) of the Neurosciences Institute at San Diego, have shown with out-standing electro physiological experiments that fruit flies, which have 250 000 neurons, sleep. It is rather an open question where dreaming first emerges in the phylogenetic tree. In like vein, it is interesting that Darwin avers that even insects express anger, terror, jealousy, and love by their stridulation.

Birds

In relation to intention as bespeaking an image in the mind, there is extremely interesting data on the fishing techniques of herons. Characteristics of fishing behaviour have been described in several species of heron, but a classic example is the green heron in Japan studied by Higuchi. Herons gather small objects or may collect a twig and break it into pieces. The heron will drop the twig in the water and watch intently, and when a minnow comes up to it as a possible food object, the heron will grab the minnow with a rapid neck extension. It has been seen that herons will sometimes retrieve a twig that has floated away, and then drop it in again. Another may fly to a branch overlooking a pond and drop the stick in. When a minnow comes up to it, the heron swoops down and takes the minnow on the wing. All manner of objects have been seen to be used for bait—twigs, leaves, berries, feathers, insects, and pieces of bread left around by visitors. Only a small group of the heron colony may manifest this bait fishing behaviour, and, though it is not clear how they learnt it, it is a reasonable hypothesis that some animals saw small fish attracted to pieces of bread dropped in the water by children. That is, it could be proposed that the bird has a plan, an image in the mind, deriving from observation, and this could imply thinking. Again, the behaviour would appear to meet the Turing test of delay with implication of consciousness, though experiments on distracting attention were not carried out.

Mammals

We have already discussed the matter of higher order consciousness—self awareness—in the primates, as well as in dolphins. Descriptions of deception by primates in experimental records are also suggestive of conscious processes. Darwin has discussed many aspects of behaviour of animals in *The Expression of Emotion in Man and Animals*, and in particular, emotions as reflecting conscious states. On this point Miriam Rothschild remarks that anyone doubting emotions in animals should try taking their dog to the vet for the second or third time.

On the issue of an animal having a plan, and executing a plan bespeaking an image of the world, a recent paper by Changeux and colleagues (Granon *et al.*, 2003) is most interesting. The maze exploring activity to get food in hungry mice was investigated. The context was that wild-type mice (i.e. normals) were compared with 'knock-out' mice. In the specific case the mice had the gene for the nicotinic acetylcholine receptor 'knocked out', i.e. deleted by a molecular biological technique. That is, as well as the natural acetylcholine neurotransmitter, which acts on the receptor, the receptor is responsive also to nicotine in the bloodstream. Thus, nicotine similarly excites the cells carrying this particular type of receptor (a receptor is a signal receiving mechanism). It explains something of the addictive actions of nicotine, given the function of the cells bearing this receptor.

Comparing the two types of mice—the receptor 'knocked out', or the normals (wild type) yielded a surprising result. In relation to utilization of memory and motivation for food it turned out, surprisingly, that the 'knock-out' animals in a maze situation were faster in getting to the goal of food than the normal animals. The cells carrying the receptor involve the prefrontal and cingulate cortices. The cells of these regions are revealed by lesion studies in rats to underpin much of the executive functions. These include exploratory functions, the balance between different components of displacements, and the succession and duration of contacts between members of the same species (conspecies). It turned out from an open field type of behaviour analysis followed on a computer that the wild-type mice showed spontaneous flexibility, and their longer time in getting to the food goal reflected time spent in exploring the environment, including objects placed there. This putative curiosity was paralleled in experiments involving contrived meeting with a conspecific. The 'knock-out' mice were rigid and did not modify their routine behaviour. They initiated approach in an exaggerated fashion and rarely started escape behaviour, whereas the normals alternated between approach and escape.

Overall, Changeux and colleagues suggest the data indicate the mice do far more than simply react to sensory information. They engage in complex extended behaviours geared towards far removed goals. They use processes that override or differentially select routines, and orchestrate locomotor behaviours according to intentions and plans—consonant with the statements of Christopher Longuet-Higgins (Kenny 1973), J.Z. Young (1986), and Christof Koch (2004) at the outset of this chapter. The investigators suggest that the 'knock-out' animals with consequent impairment of function, in particular, of prefrontal and cingulate cortices, reproduce some of the impairments seen in autism, and attention-deficit hyperactivity disorders. Certain types of nicotinic acid receptors are reduced in the frontal cortex in such clinical cases, and nicotine administration may improve the clinical condition.

Overview of some aspects of evolution of the vertebrate brain and cognitive processes

An overview that embodies both the consideration of comparative data and the intuition of many scientists of its implication is stated by Stephen Walker (1983). He points to the incontrovertible fact that evolution has entrained increased complexity in both animals and plants. However, it is difficult to decide which species are more primitive and which are more advanced in particular regards. The branching in the phylogenetic tree can be discerned, and the brains of higher vertebrates are much bigger than those of lower vertebrates, and perhaps, better. However, they can be described in terms of their main subdivisions—hindbrain, midbrain, and forebrain. The forebrain has expanded most with time and this is evident with humans, with the forebrain predominant for intelligence, thought and cognition. Hannah Damassio and colleagues report that the frontal lobe as a percentage of the hemisphere volume is 28.1 in the macaque, and 37.1 in the human. This represents a large augmentation of the possible neuronal connections of the frontal lobe in humans, which could subserve a neuronal global workspace to be discussed in Chapter 11.

Walker (1983) supports the idea that the function of different parts of the brain may be similar in all vertebrates, and there might be expectation that the higher psychological functions in animals might be related to how far the forebrain has developed. Fish, frogs, and lizards do not have much in the way of cerebral hemispheres, and thus, not much in the way of cognition could be expected. However, this is more generous than some other viewpoints, which regard the presence of the forebrain in such creatures as a response system to smells, or to programme primitive instincts as distinct from serving cognition, learning, or attention. He feels this is probably wrong because the cerebral hemispheres of lower vertebrates share several anatomical and physiological characteristics with the cerebral hemispheres of mammals. Further, the units, the neurons, are basically similar in vertebrate species. Therefore, the hemispheres of lower vertebrates should have some psychological functions in common with the forebrain of mammals. Functions emergent may be difficult to delineate, but perhaps functions such as emotions, plans of action, goals and values, and selective direction of perception seem to require the higher levels of brain function.

Ethology or comparative behaviour studies

The clear difference between impetus to gratification and biological purpose

The strict behaviourists have earned some credit for championing a discipline of analysis of behaviour that did avoid crude anthropomorphism—seeing animal behaviour through human eyes. The demise of behaviourism as a dominant dictate was a result of several trends. Actually, psychologists, psychoanalysts, and like disciplines ignored it. The discipline of ethology (comparative behaviour) did much to dispel it. This approach was to a considerable extent driven by European students concerned with instinctive behaviour and with observation of what animals actually did in their natural circumstances. Whereas, their descriptions do not often invoke conscious processes as a pivotal explanation of what happens, the terminology they used for crucial ideas is clearly directed to brain processes determinant of what the animal is seen to do.

Thus, as said earlier, the increasing readiness of an animal to engage in an instinctive repertoire of action is characterized by the build up of 'action specific energy' in the brain. In order to make the concept explicable to the reader, Konrad Lorenz (1950), for example, used the analogy of a reservoir filling up, as various processes within the organism and brain (e.g. hormone secretion) contrive particular conditions in the brain. These give a very strong readiness to carry out the instinctive behaviour pattern concerned. The organism, as it were, is ready to go 'pop' in the face of presentation of a particular stimulus, which is the one genetically apt to set in motion the instinctive behaviour concerned—it is the 'innate releasing mechanism'. Indeed, one phenomenon embodied in the ethological description is termed 'the vacuum pattern'. This is the circumstance where the propensity to embark on an instinctive behaviour pattern is very high. However, there is an absence of stimuli of the innate releasing mechanism. The animal shows 'intention movements', which are partial behaviours appropriate to the beginning of the instinctive repertoire. They can be considered diagnostic of a high state of central excitation. The behaviour in which the endogenous energy is finally discharged was called 'consummatory action', which is the motor part of the innate behaviour.

Tinbergen (1951) has given a masterly analysis of these phenomena in his book *The Study of Instinct*. This text provides a compelling outline of the complexity of the behaviour patterns of many species, and how neural systems subserving them often unfold in staged fashion with development of the animal, and become correspondingly more sensitive to internal influences such as hormone secretions.

A main force behind the emergence of the comparative study of behaviour was in continental Europe and was led by Niko Tinbergen, Konrad Lorenz, and von Frisch. [The discipline had, however, many historical antecedents, which they cite extensively in their writings (Whitman, von Uexhüll, Heinroth, and others). There were also major scholars in this area in the United Kingdom, including W.H. Thorpe, Robert Hinde, and Patrick Bateson of Cambridge, who contributed both original observation and conceptual analysis.]

Lorenz, himself, paid a great tribute to Wallace Craig of the USA, who contributed a major insight into the determination of animal and, thus, human behaviour. He sets the impact of Craig's insight against the background of the dispute between 'vitalists' and 'mechanists'.

As Lorenz puts it, vitalists base their arguments on a dogmatic assertion that all life processes are governed by an essentially non-explainable, beyond the natural, directing vital force. Mechanists replied that all life processes could be explained eventually on the foundations of the laws of physics. Organic systems could be explained on the basis of a sum of the elements. He notes that antagonistic exaggerations of the two schools had a deleterious effect on the scientific study of behaviour.

It is undeniable that animal behaviour in most cases develops a definite survival value. It is directed towards a particular purpose. This survival value and purpose did not seem to vitalistic thinkers to offer problems. Indeed, 'instinct' and 'purpose', as it were, got spelled by them in capital letters, and were regarded as directly following the non-explainable directive factor of life.

Along with other instances, Lorenz (1950) notes that whether an animal is striving to obtain some end or goal and changing its behaviour adaptively to reach it, or a stereotyped behaviour pattern automatically develops some survival value, the directive factor is telling the organism what to do. This is as it appears in the eyes of the purposive psychologists.

It is, therefore, only consistent to identify the survival value of any kind of innate behaviour patterns with the end or goal at which the organism is aiming.

Now, the salient point of Lorenz (1950) is as follows—He says that it was Wallace Craig who cleared up this confused thinking. *Craig once and for all, exploded the myth of the 'infallability' of instinct.* He did so with a wealth of observation, by showing the animal is not aiming at the survival value of its activities, but essentially at the discharge of certain actions. He termed it consummatory action. *Lorenz says the recognition of this indubitable fact is one of the utter commonplaces that are so amazingly hard to discover.* Essentially there are three successive stages in innate behaviour.

1 Accumulation of action specific energy giving rise to *appetitive behaviour.*

2 Appetitive behaviour striving for, seeking and attaining a stimulus situation which activates the *innate releasing mechanism.*

3 Setting the releasing mechanism in action with discharge of the endogenous energy in a *consummatory action.*

Introspection makes it transparently obvious that the purpose of Wallace Craig's appetitive behaviour is the discharge of the instinctive action, and not its survival value. *It is the gratification of an instinctively generated appetite by a consummatory act—not its biological purpose.* In a water-deprived animal or human the consummatory act of drinking is to gratify or satisfy thirst. It is not any perceived purpose to reduce a high salt concentration of the blood or repair a reduced plasma volume, which conjointly engendered the thirst. In the same way one does not eat in order to rectify a lowered blood glucose concentration, or to stop stomach contractions that conjointly may be contributing to the genesis of the sensation of hunger. It is to satisfy a subjective desire—hunger—the desire to eat food. Lorenz (1950) says 'I eat though it is my purpose to lose weight.' Similarly, at the extreme, though breathlessness is caused by an increased carbon dioxide concentration in the blood, the animal or human does not gasp for air—fight for air—to reduce the carbon dioxide concentration in the blood. As Lorenz puts it—'Desire for gratification is in the chair, so to speak, and makes the human or creature do it, though the action has an unequivocal survival value.'

He says that, *however obvious and even commonplace Wallace Craig's discovery may seem, it was undoubtedly one of the most decisive steps forward towards a real understanding of behaviour.*

In a biological overview it is equivalently clear that these considerations apply to the process of reproduction. The animal inhabitants of the earth (including usually the human species notwithstanding some religious dogma to the contrary) do not engage in sexual intercourse with the aim of increasing their numbers—of producing little members of their species. This is obvious from contemplating a group of dogs around a female dog on heat. Their intention, their consummatory act is not governed by the dim concept that it would be nice to have some puppies. The dogs are squabbling over which one shall have the gratification of mounting the female.

Jaak Panksepp (1998) has stated 'It is a remarkable feat of nature to weave powerful sexual feelings and desire in the fabric of the brain without revealing the reproductive purpose of those feelings to the eager participants.'

Chapter 5

The appetite for salt and the mind: intention in salt mining elephants

This chapter sets the behaviour of a large mammal against the four statements made at the beginning of Chapter 4. The account to follow may be considered an exemplar of intention of an animal directed to an object not immediately present—an issue emphasized by J.Z. Young.

Mount Elgon in Kenya

High on an extinct volcano in tropical Africa, just 1° north of the Equator, a quite unique and remarkable biological event occurs. It involves elephants trekking long distances to a goal. They go into a large cave in complete darkness to mine and eat salt.

Mount Elgon, an extinct volcano on the Kenya/Uganda border, has a ring of peaks around a central caldera about 8 km in diameter. The highest peak reaches 4321 metres (14.178 ft). The diameter of the mountain at its base is about 95 km (60 miles). The slopes of the mountain are covered by dense rain forest up to about 2600 metres. Then the rain forest is replaced by thick stands of bamboo, and then by Afro-Alpine vegetation including the strange looking giant lobelias. It is about 3–4 million years since Mount Elgon erupted, but it is still the site of geothermal activity, with hot springs with temperature at 49°C. The Mount Elgon National Park is situated on the eastern slope of the mountain. Mount Elgon is part of the geological events involving the 5000 km (3000) mile) African–Arabian Rift Valley system, which was a series of parallel faults stretching from Mozambique via the Red Sea to the Valley of Jordan. The basic event was the upthrust of the whole of East Africa by pressure under the earth's crust resulting in volcanoes, and long flat-bottomed valleys.

This region is the locale of the event, unique in the world, of the 5 ton mammal, the elephant, going deep underground in pitch blackness to mine and eat salt.

The major credit for the study of this remarkable behaviour and description of its setting rests with Ian Redmond, a British biologist from Bristol. Also,

Anthony Sutcliffe of the British Museum, and others have been important contributors. When the various implications in relation to brain mechanisms and the cultural organization of elephant society are addressed, issues of fundamental importance emerge.

Formation of caves on Mount Elgon

Ian Redmond (1982, 1985) reports elephants visited the two caves he studied (Kitum and Makingeny) singly or in groups of up to 19, and the visits usually began about dusk and lasted up to 6 hours. Herbivorous animals and monkeys, rodents, carnivores, bats, and baboons visited the caves as did the local cattle farmers. The motive of the carnivores may have reflected that it was an advantageous place to prey on herbivores. The herbivores needed salt, as will be explained. The carnivores needed the herbivores.

As Redmond describes, the mode of formation of Mount Elgon was principally explosive, with huge quantities of lava boulders, volcanic ash, and dust being thrown out over the surrounding area to form a volcanic agglomerate, which is much in evidence in outcrops today. This material is occasionally imbedded with lava flows, which came in the final stages of Elgon's volcanic activity, and these cooled to become erosion-resistant layers of basalt-like rock. Most of the caves are found beneath the tip formed by the leading downhill edge of lava flow. In the caves are the petrified trunks of trees felled by the blast. The caves are mostly variants of the same theme with a cul-de-sac extending into the hillside from a cliff. Sometimes fallen rock, as a result of collapse of the overhang, obstructs the access. The presence of a waterfall cascading over the cave mouth suggests that salt mining may have begun where rock underlying the lava edge was softened by splashing water.

Redmond thinks these large caves were excavated by elephants who have been eating the mineral-rich rocks for tens of thousands, maybe hundreds of thousands of years. The volume of Kitum Cave is something like 20–40 million litres, and on this basis, if 1 litre of rock per week were ingested it would take 500 000 to 1 000 000 years, but this is a very low estimate of the rate of ingestion and the time could be less.

Kitum cave has a 'letter box' type entrance about 40 metres wide. The cave extends into the mountain for 160 metres. Inside it widens to about 100 metres, and a cul de sac with interior walls, which have been excavated by years of mining activity. Elephants tusk directly at the cave wall and also at the broken rock fragments on the cave floor, which they pick up and eat. These fragments are often covered by salt crusts. The temperature of the cave remains constant at night at 13.5°C so it is much warmer than the outside mountain. The elephants may remain in there most of the night to keep warm. As well as tusking and eating the salt rock, they play, bath, or rub on the rocks. Redmond has spent many nights in the caves with the elephants who have come to accept his presence despite flashlight photographs. A film unit of Channel 4 UK has made a remarkable movie of the elephants in action in the caves.

The analysis of rocks and encrustations on their surface show they are rich in sodium, calcium and magnesium. Sodium is present as sodium chloride, sodium carbonate, and sodium sulphate. Of other biologically relevant ions, phosphate and iron are also present. The sodium content of the rocks is over 100 times the sodium content of the vegetation in the surrounding forest.

The elephants cannot lick rock as their tongues aren't long enough, so they loosen earth or gouge off bits of rock with their tusks and then transfer the lumps to their mouth with the trunk, and grind them with their molars. During their lifetime, elephants have progressively six sets of molars and eating rocks may wear these down more rapidly, and thus may shorten their life expectancy. However, the most conspicuous effect is that the tusks of the elephants in the region are worn down to the extent that they may become short rounded stumps.

Many studies show that elephants will seek out salt sources and licks in various parts of Africa. Weir (1972) has shown in the Wankie National Park in Zimbabwe that the population density of elephants in various regions is directly related to the salt content of the available water, being highest where salt content is highest. The density is not related to the abundance of herbage. Elephants are observed to excavate in sand and soil to find licks. The National Geographic magazine has recently reported in three editions the extraordinary trek by Dr Fay across the Congo and Gabon, an ecological study involving over a year of walking in primeval jungle. He and colleagues recount in the Congo National Parks a thinning of forest areas dotted around the region where elephants and game seek salt along the river banks. Gorillas are also abundant there. Dr Carolyn Tutin, her colleagues, and I, have observed active use of salt licks in the Lope National Park in the Gabon, and have made cafeteria experiments with soil impregnated with different salts, and have shown, *inter alia*, intake of NaCl impregnated soil by elephants.

However, the underground salt mining in the Mount Elgon National Park is unique in the world. Redmond believes the knowledge of the caves and their mineral content is passed down from elephant to elephant through generations, from mother to calf. In this sense it is cultural transmission of knowledge.

Elephant behaviour within the caves

Redmond writes,

> Picture yourself on a ledge in a cave mouth with a waterfall splashing on moss-covered rocks. Suddenly the moonlit forest vibrates with a deep elephantine rumble. The miners are here. Slowly and cautiously, trunks snaking at the whiff of a human, they pace in single file along the familiar trail and up the steep entrance path. Then, one by one, they disappear into the deeper gloom of Kitum cave.

Family herds would walk in line, trunk to tail like circus elephants to avoid any youngsters straying into danger (Fig. 5.1).

Once the elephants become accustomed to a tame human moving about the rocks they would tolerate his presence in the cave. Redmond could climb on rocks inside the vast cave and look along a flashlight beam to make his observations. He watched elephants feeling their way around boulders bigger than themselves, splashing through pools, the cows keeping a protective trunk on the calves, and with fruit bats swinging free on their roost, and circling overhead. Redmond says 'the adults knew, I am sure, that the crevasse in the old pile of fallen rock claimed the lives of at least two calves and several antelope.

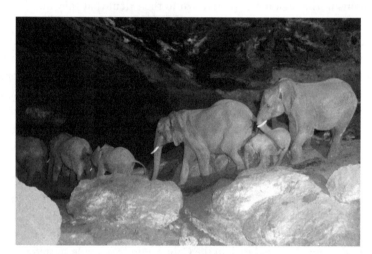

Figure 5.1 Elephants photographed by Dr Ian Redmond in Kitum Cave on Mount Elgon in Kenya. The salt hungry animals go 100 metres in pitch darkness to gouge out the sodium sulphate rock on the walls of the cave. This behaviour has most likely been going on for tens of thousands of years, in as far as the size of the cave reflects the mining behaviour of the elephants. Redmond suggests that the knowledge of the topography of the caves and their mineral content is a cultural transmission from generation to generation.

See also Colour Plate 15.

One wrong foot in the dark would mean a slow agonizing death. Once past the crevasse the elephants would spread out across the back chamber and begin mining.'

Redmond remarks that as the elephants came to accept his presence, so he came to respect their remarkable intelligence. He has been impressed by the way a baby elephant learns from its parents and elders where to find food, water, and salt. This knowledge is passed down from generation to generation, and each population of elephants benefits from the accumulated wisdom of its forebears. In human tribes we refer to this as a culture. The use of caves on Mount Elgon is a feature of Elgon elephant culture and accounts for their relaxed behaviour underground.

The clunk and thud of tusk on rock would be followed by the amazing harsh sound of molars crunching and grinding on rock. The back of the cave is so dark that even during the day you cannot see your hand in front of your face. Presumptively the same would apply to an elephant seeing its trunk. Most visits took place after dark and could last for hours on end.

Television cameras with infra-red light and image intensifier caught a cow throwing dust over herself, another suckling a calf and one night two teenage bulls were seen play-fighting and sparring. Some time there is spent sleeping. Redmond notes that the decisions in a family of elephants are made by the matriarch, and she decides when to leave. Her sisters, daughters, and offspring may be spread out all over the cave snoozing, splashing in pools, or mining. Usually there was a stunning roar, filling the cave with solid sound, and after this in the silence, the sound of elephant hides rubbing together, and a splash of footsteps, as elephants gathered prior to climbing over the mound of old roof fall. This was the dangerous bit, avoiding the crevasse again, yet he saw a large cow, the matriarch he presumed, shoving and butting a younger elephant into the lead position. Was she ensuring her offspring learnt the layout of the cave? He had a distinct impression that the elephant miners had some sort of mental map of the cave layout much the same way as blind people become familiar with the location of furniture and local amenities. On one occasion he watched a confident young bull on the way out, he speeded up as he climbed on to the mound, casting his trunk forward every couple of steps as if making sure of a path he already knew.

In observing mining of an individual elephant, Redmond estimated the amount of rock he consumed during a visit amounted to a gallon bucket full—about 4–5 litres in volume. Based on the sodium content of the rock analyses reported by Redmond and his colleagues, Bowell and Warren, a rough estimate of intake could range up to 20 g of sodium per kilogram of rock eaten, which would be a very significant amount physiologically (i.e. 80–100 g of sodium—about 1–2% of body sodium content). A litre of blood plasma contains about 3.5 g of sodium, or 9 g of salt. Possibly a visit every 5–10 days would keep them near salt replete.

Slaughter of the elephants

The elephants pay a high price for their salt intake. The mining wears down the ivory of their tusks faster than it can grow, and the Elgon elephants have stumpy tusks that just protrude beyond the base of the trunk, and yet the high price of ivory in the 1980s led to heavy poaching. Despite the fact that the worn tusks would be a compromise as a source, the poachers used small calibre machine guns and simply sprayed the herds with bullets. The tusks were cut off as part of the face with chain saws. The area, including the approach to Kitum cave became full of the stench of rotting flesh (Redmond 1987). Numbers were reduced from 1100 down to perhaps no more than 100 animals, and the Mount Elgon National Park was closed while the rangers, with help from the army, captured 11 poachers, and to a considerable extent stopped the process. The world banned the ivory trade but some poaching still goes on to supply the market among mindless wealthy people for ivory trinkets and bangles. Several elephants were killed in 1990 and one ranger was killed. Redmond launched an appeal to set up an African Ele Fund and donations to the Born Free Foundation have been diverted to this source to support repair of patrol vehicles and equipment, and to monitor elephant populations and counter and capture poachers who come from Uganda and Kenya.

Why do the elephants become salt deficient and seek it?

In a book, *The Hunger for Salt: An anthropological, physiological and medical analysis* (Denton, 1982), I have set out the biological basis of the answer to this question.

In the absence of geological sources of salt, rainwater is the main source of salt in the soil and vegetation of the planet, and therefore, for herbivorous animals. Winds carry marine aerosols inland, and as distance increases from the seas and oceans that surround the land, the amount of salt in rainwater decreases. By 150–200 km inland, the salt in rainwater is near that of distilled water. This was discovered by Swedish and Australian meteorologists. It is the reason why the interior of continents and alpine areas are salt deficient.

Take the alpine areas of Australia as an example. In the Snowy Mountains in south-east Australia during the spring and early summer the grass has only about 1–2% of the salt (sodium) content that the coastal grass has. A kilogram of mountain grass has only about one-hundredth of the salt content of a litre of blood plasma. In chemical terms, a kilogram of grass contains 1 mmol of sodium. To give a quantitative slant to this level in the mountain grass, the presently recommended sodium intake for the US population is 100 mmol/day—that is the sodium content of 100 kilograms (220 pounds weight) of this mountain grass. Very low levels of sodium are also characteristic of the grass in central Australia, which receives rain from the annual monsoons from the north—the coast may be a thousand kilometres or more distant. Essentially, the same is true in the great Amazon basin, where sodium content of rain and river water is minute—approaching trace metal levels. In inland continental North America, the Rocky Mountains, and also in large parts of Africa—particularly in the equatorial rain forest regions, the same situation holds. The heavy rainfall of tropical jungle regions of Africa and South America would also work to leach out any sodium already present in soil.

In the alpine areas in the world, the freezing and thawing of soil would break it up and increase the effect of rain in leaching out any sodium present in it. Apart from some interesting plants with a particular ability to accumulate sodium from the impoverished soil, most of the vegetation, like the soil, is very low in salt.

The herbivorous creatures, the grass eaters, comprising the game animals of the earth as well as the grazing pastoral animals, bear the major impact of the salt-deficient ecosystem, which means very large areas of the continents. Salt lack, however, also occurs in omnivores, such as primates and rodents, as well as in humans.

The carnivorous animals do not face this deficiency problem because there is always adequate sodium in the muscle tissue, viscera, and blood of their prey. In fact there is about 50 mmol/kg wet-weight in muscle and viscera, which represents about 3 g of sodium chloride per kilogram eaten. For comparison blood plasma has 150 mmol per kg or litre which amounts to 8.7 grams of sodium chloride per kilogram or litre.

The colonization during evolution of the salt and/or water impoverished ecosystems of the planet. Body fluid regulation and the emergence of intention

The scarcity of salt in very large areas of the earth, as well as the fact that fresh water also may be in short supply, highlights in striking manner the problems of regulation of body fluids. Keeping both the composition and the volume of body fluids constant was a necessary condition for the emergence of life on dry land. During evolution, progressively more intricate and sensitive mechanisms developed. Indeed, one of the paramount insights in the history of physiological science was that of the French genius Claude Bernard (1957) who stated 'The stability of the miliéu interiéur is the primary condition for freedom and independence of existence; the mechanism which allows this is that which ensures in the miliéu interiéur the maintenance of all the conditions necessary to the life of the elements.' (miliéu interiéur = the body fluids.)

To put this in evolutionary context, following the development of the single cell organisms from earlier life forms, there followed the emergence of multicellular organisms. These had tissues with special functions. Organs such as the liver, brain, muscles, and digestive tract involved aggregates of millions of cells. The development of a closed circulation system with pumping by the heart allowed the circulation of fluids around the cells of these special tissues. The tissue fluids carried nutrients to the cells deep in the mass of the specialized organ and took away the waste products produced by the cells. A single cell carries out these functions through its surface, but once millions of cells had gathered as a special organ, an organized circulation of tissue fluids as a result of the pumping heart became essential.

The ancient ocean

The pattern of chemicals of the tissue fluid and blood plasma (the circulating miliéu interiéur of Claude Bernard), which developed, and was perpetuated in creatures evolving later on, embodied the chemical composition of the ancient ocean at the time, some 500 million years or more ago, when this closed circulation system of the metazoa, or many celled organisms, first evolved.

The pattern of ions—the ratio of one to the other (that is, sodium, potassium, calcium magnesium, chloride, bicarbonate, phosphate) is broadly similar in fish, amphibians, reptiles, monotremes (platypus), birds, marsupials, and mammals (Table 5.1). When the first backboned fishes invaded the freshwater rivers created by mountain uplift during the Ordovician geological period about 400 million years ago, they faced a major chemical problem. No longer did the composition of the surrounding watery medium largely correspond to the ionic patterns and concentration of their internal circulating tissue fluids. Fresh river water (water free of the oceanic salts) could enter their bodies through their skin, and also from the gut when water was swallowed in the course of feeding. This threatened to dilute the body fluids circulating around cells.

Here it needs to be explained that individual cells have a semipermeable membrane surrounding them. This encloses the nucleus that has the genetic material, and also the cytoplasm, which is composed of water, dissolved salts, proteins, and many organelles with different functions. In particular, there are the mitochondria that serve energy generation. Water can move in and out of cells in accordance with the concentration of dissolved particles on either side of the membrane. In this case of flux of fresh water into the body and tissue fluids, the dissolved particles inside the cells would draw water from the tissue fluids into the cells and they would swell. This would disrupt the chemical and electrical processes, which are the basis of the normal function of cells. At the geological time when this chemical challenge caused by freshwater rivers began, the crucial evolutionary step was the emergence of the kidney equipped with glomeruli. That is, a kidney that passed the blood through a million little filters. It continuously excreted the excess water as well as the waste products of metabolism. Also, with its system of long kidney tubules it jealously extracted from the filtrate and transported back into the blood the precious salts and nutrients of the blood and tissue fluid circulatory system. So they were not lost—only the water and waste products became urine. Scales, together with secretions, which made the skin impermeable to water, also helped to stop fresh water entering the animal.

Table 5.1 Composition of Blood Plasma of Various Species of Animals. The similarity of the pattern across the evolutionary tree is evident

Animal	Na	K	Ca	Mg	Cl	HCO₃
	Plasma concentration mmol/litre					
Lamprey	120	3.2	2.0	2.1	96	6.4
Shark	200	8.2	3.0	2.0	181	6.0
Brown Trout	142	3.5	3.4	1.9	123	7.0
Sea Trout	166	3.5	3.4	–	138	11.0
Frog	104	2.5	2.0	1.2	74	25
Iguana	157	3.5	2.7	0.9	118	24
Chicken	154	6.0	5.6	2.3	122	
Sperm Whale	170	2.6	0.2	2.3	120	

(From J.T. Fitzsimons, "The Physiology of Thirst and Sodium Appetite", Cambridge University Press, 1979)

Animal	Na	K	Ca	Mg	Cl	
Platypus	165	3.5	5.0	1.7	128	
Spiny Ant eater	139	5.0	5.6	0.9	104	
RatKangaroo	149	4.6	4.4	2.0	107	
Koala	144	3.6	4.8	3.0	105	
Wombat	138	5.8	5.2	2.1	97	
Black-tailed Wallaby	143	4.8	5.2	1.7	99	
Sheep	157	4.9	4.2	0.7	106	
Human	143	4.5	4.5	2.0	105	

Plasma composition of Australian animals compared with human. *(From Denton, Wynn, McDonald and Simon, Acta Medica Scandinavica, 140: Supp. 261, 1–202, 1951)*

As life evolved further and amphibians and reptiles migrated from the swamps on to dry land, the regulatory problems became greater and different.

The evolution of systems to deal with them was a necessary condition for the remarkable colonization of the earth's surface by diverse species of animals. The colonization culminated eventually with the emergence of the mammals. The new environmentally determined dangers were shortage of water, and often shortage of salt, the main chemical of the circulating blood and tissue fluids. The overruling necessity was to have a near constant water content of the body to sustain the circulatory system and the numerous and versatile metabolic processes. Two masterpieces of evolutionary invention emerged with the colonization of dry land. They reflect the genesis of intentional behaviour.

Thirst

First there was the development of the thirst system, a neural organization in the brain engendering a primal emotion that causes intention to seek and drink water if it is needed. Water is lost constantly as a result of water vapour lost with breathing. It is lost through the skin, and also as a result of the formation of urine to excrete waste products. It has to be replaced. This need, giving rise to thirst, is signalled by brain sensors responding to the fact that the salt concentration of the blood rises if replacement of water lost is inadequate. Also a separate set of messages from sensors that measure stretch and thus filling of the vessels of the circulation can signal that decrease of the volume of fluid in the circulation has occurred. Separate neural pathways from these sensors on vessels feed to the brain and they also generate thirst. (In a way, this gave a double security. For example, fluid lost from the body may contain salts, as with sweating. The salt concentration of sweat is less than that in blood, so even though the loss represented water in excess of salt, the change in blood plasma sodium would not be as great as would occur if pure water was lost as occurs from the lungs. However, the volume of water lost would be as great, so the alternate line of defence depending on volume is an advantage.)

A second and complementary mechanism of water regulation is the operation of a hormone system to help conserve water by restricting loss from the kidney. The concentration of this specific hormone in the blood that facilitates water conservation by the kidney increases as the salt concentration in the blood rises. This hormone is called the antidiuretic hormone or vasopressin. It is secreted by the pituitary gland (a small gland at the base of the brain). Its secretion is regulated by sensors in the hypothalamus in the base of the brain. They respond to the salt concentration of the blood. There are also stretch receptors in the vessels, which respond to the volume of blood in the circulatory system. However, as loss of water from the body is continuous, this system can only act to reduce loss via the kidney. It cannot replace water. Only thirst and drinking does this.

Salt appetite

The other side of the coin, was the problem of keeping constant the salt content of the circulating fluids of the body. This was in the face of the fact that salt intake from food in large parts of the planet could be very low. Salt loss could occur in urine. In different species of animals salt loss occurs also in the course of keeping temperature constant. This salt is lost in sweat, by drooling saliva when respiration is used to control temperature, and also when animals put saliva, which contains salt, on their skin and fur to cause evaporative cooling. Obviously, salt loss in body temperature control can be made greater by disease states that cause fever. Salt loss in temperature control becomes greater if active exercise is involved.

Conservation of salt is achieved by the salt retaining hormone, aldosterone, which is secreted by the adrenal gland—a structure in the abdomen just above the kidney. Its secretion into the blood acts on the kidney to conserve salt and also it reduces the sodium content of the sweat and gut secretions. The secretion of this hormone increases appropriately when the salt content of the body is decreasing. Obviously, if the salt content of food is very low, the animal is much more vulnerable to environmental conditions that cause depletion of salt.

Again, it is evident that, whereas salt retention under the aegis of aldosterone is important, a mechanism to increase intake in the face of depletion is essential.

Now, in tandem with the evolution of a kidney able to retain salt, there developed brain mechanisms that generated a hunger for salt when the body was depleted of this substance. Salt was crucial to the integrity of the circulation. A normal concentration of salt (the sodium cation) in tissue fluids is very important also for normal function of specialized tissues, including nerve cells. When the body is deficient of salt, the volume of blood and tissue fluids decreases. Blood pressure falls and the capacity of the creature to fight, to flee, or range over large territories for food decreases. An extreme instance causing this situation is infectious disease of the type that causes diarrhoea. This effectively kills humans, and has been recorded as a cause of death of great apes in the wild. The worst example in humans is cholera, where huge amounts of salt and water are lost. The individual may die rapidly as a result of collapse of the circulation.

The actual chemical mechanisms in the neurons of the brain, which generate the specific craving for salt, involve fascinating and complex events. These happen in special brain cells, which are dedicated to creating this specific appetite. That is, these cells in the basal part of the brain called the hypothalamus are the nub of detection of salt deficiency. They set alight a whole genetically wired network of nerve cells, which contrive a desire or appetite to seek, find, and ingest salt.

The ignition of this system may come from decrease of salt, that is, the sodium concentration of the blood. However, as with thirst, it comes from decrease in the volume of the circulation. This change in the volume of blood in the great vessels activates a complex hormone system called the renin–angiotensin system. The hormone angiotensin is the product of a cascade of chemical reactions that begin with the enzyme renin produced in the kidney, which acts on the precursor of angiotensin, which is called angiotensinogen and is produced in the liver. Angiotensin is intimately involved in brain actions within the nerve cell systems, which subserve salt appetite and help to generate it. We will describe this further on.

Validation of sodium deficiency in wild animals

To make a complete analysis of the elephants' behaviour, it would be ideal if it were possible to obtain specimens of blood, urine, salivary secretion, and tissue to show that at the times the elephants visited the caves to seek salt they were indeed showing signs of sodium deficiency, whereas at other times they were not. Such information has been obtained from other species of wild animals visiting salt licks in other parts of the world.

In the Snowy Mountains of Australia, a salt-deficient region where the sodium content of grass is extremely low in spring and early summer as recorded earlier in this chapter, it has been shown that kangaroos and introduced species of animals such as wild rabbits, have high blood levels of the salt-retaining hormone aldosterone, and high levels of the hormone renin, which stimulates the secretion of aldosterone. When sodium deficiency occurs the production of angiotensin caused by renin acts on the outer layer of the adrenal gland to cause secretion of aldosterone as well as having an action in the brain as referred to above. The animals have little or no sodium (salt) in the urine. This is at the time when they show an avid appetite for any source of salt. Moreover, the outer rim of the adrenal gland, which secretes the salt-retaining hormone, is very greatly enlarged and the duct system of the salivary glands is radically changed because the cellular layer, the epithelium, which transports ions, is enlarged. This reflects the fact that herbivores secrete very large volumes of saliva. A cow, for example, secretes 20–40 litres of saliva per day and as they become salt depleted, they conserve salt by reducing the sodium content of their salivary secretion and substitute potassium for it. Potassium is readily available from the grass that they digest, so it is a brilliant physiological adaptation. It allows the really copious volume of salivary secretion, which makes digestion in ruminants feasible to continue and not be stopped because of the limited sodium supply of the body. This saliva is pooled in the capacious rumen of the foregut where digestion occurs.

The large volume of salivary secretion, which is normally made up of sodium bicarbonate and sodium phosphate, gives a fluid medium in which the rich flora of microorganisms that digest the cellulose of grass and herbage can flourish. If it were not for this change of composition, feasible because of the abundant supply of potassium from grass, the animal would have to draw on the sodium in its circulating blood and tissue fluids and bone to keep digestion going. This would compromise its blood pressure and tissue nutrition. The change in the architecture of the salivary glands noted, reflects this change in the secretory ion transport mechanism involving substitution of potassium for sodium in the copious saliva.

In fact, this mechanism of coping with salt deficiency (a large change in the ratio of sodium to potassium in saliva), which I discovered in herbivores at the Howard Florey Institute in Australia, has been an adaptation of paramount survival value in evolution; for on it has depended the ability of herbivorous ruminating animals—the wild game and pastoral animals—to colonize the very extensive sodium deficient areas of the planet. It complements the evolution of the brain mechanism generating a specific appetite for salt (Fig. 5.2).

So, direct studies in other parts of the world, have shown that it is very likely the elephants of the tropical jungle around Mount Elgon are salt deficient, and oscillate on the edge of this metabolic situation, and episodically repair the deficit by a visit to the caves. The specificity of the appetite they show, and the rock analyses would seem to confirm this.

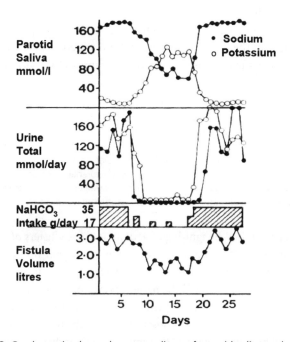

Figure 5.2 Grazing animals produce many litres of parotid saliva each day to assist in the digestion. Here one of the two parotid ducts of a sheep has been exteriorised surgically so the salivary flow is lost from the body and collected (about 3 litres/day). Each day the animal has been given 35g sodium bicarbonate to replace the sodium lost. When this supplement is stopped the animal becomes deficient in salt. The sodium content of the saliva decreases and the potassium concentration increases. They decrease to negligible level in the urine. They are conserved. In effect, the animal has used the potassium content of grass to run its digestive system. The creature is able to carry on digestion exactly as in nature when the salt content of grass is negligible. This happens in the interior of continents and in the mountains. The salt retaining hormone of the adrenal gland controls this process.

It is obvious that some wonderfully interesting data on how well the elephants are doing in their management of their sodium balance could be acquired by darting with anaesthetic syringes in the wild using short-acting anaesthetic and with collection of blood from ear veins, as well as saliva and urine. It would, however, be somewhat dangerous. Extensive laboratory studies of the evocation of salt appetite in animals have shown the close correlation of blood chemistry with behaviour when salt replete and salt deficient. The elephants themselves would seem to provide the answer by their behaviour. As noted earlier, the rabbits, kangaroos, sheep, and cattle in the Alps of Australia, exhibit avid salt appetite. The characteristic blood and tissue chemical changes of sodium deficiency were found in spring and early summer at the time salt appetite was manifest.

Aldosterone and angiotensin can together act on the salt appetite-generating neural system in the brain to increase sodium appetite as we have shown in baboons, as does the decrease of sodium concentration of brain fluids in ruminants.

Angiotensin concentration is increased in the blood when salt is lacking, and the deficiency state also causes it to be produced locally in the brain. All of these changes would entrain alteration in the chemical status and the electrical firing of the specific groupings of nerve cells in a region in the base of the brain, the hypothalamus. Not all aspects of chemical interaction and locality of neuronal groups involved are yet understood, but a population of neurons specifically subserves and reacts to change of body salt status. There are areas in the hypothalamus, which when stimulated electrically cause an animal to selectively drink a salt solution—i.e. it chooses it in preference to water.

It can be proposed that the igniting of activity in these clusters of hypothalamic cell groups sets off excitation in other regions higher up in the brain, specifically the evolutionary ancient cerebral cortex of the brain. This includes the cingulate gyrus, the insula and the parahippocampus. Firing up activity in these cortical regions conjoint with the primary hypothalamic excitation, changes the stream of the animal's consciousness by the invasion of a hunger for salt. It should be noted, however, that my statement indicting these regions in the process is still conjectural; inferred from human brain imaging, which shows these areas of the evolutionary ancient brain cortex respond to thirst and hunger for food.

When such a primal emotion or desire becomes operative in the elephants, the most salient accompanying neural event probably would be the excitation of a hippocampal encoded memory of the location of the rich source of salt in the cave. (Hippocampus—a portion of the temporal lobe of the brain that subserves memory.) Thus, one or more members would lead the herd on a trek through the jungle to the mountain and its cave—a bit like W.B. Yeates' poem 'And I will rise, now, and go to Innisfree'. The memory would involve the whole programme of navigation in the cave in the dark, including the vital need to avoid the dangerous crevasse to reach the wall. Given the communal conditions of grazing in the jungle, many animals of the herd may reach the state of salt deficiency more or less contemporaneously. The image in the mind may occur in several animals and the matriarch or other elder is the leader to the goal.

An alternative conjecture on elephant behaviour

We could entertain an alternative idea sceptical of this hypothesis. The responses in the basal area of the brain to the chemical changes in the miliéu interiéur, which follow the progressive salt deficiency of jungle dwelling animals are hard-wired—i.e. genetically determined. The elephants might be considered essentially as automatons, and, as the specific cells at the base of the brain are excited, a general non-specific arousal of appetite occurs. The ethologists and Nobel Laureates, Konrad Lorenz (1950) and Niko Tinbergen (1951) described appetitive behaviour as the first stage of arousal and the acting out of an instinctive behavioural repertoire. This restlessness and increased random movement of the animals, as part of a general appetitive behaviour, causes them to come by chance within proximity of, for example, the Kitum cave. Sodium is the key element, and the deficiency of it causes the excitatory state in the basal brain.

In the Kitum cave one of the major sodium salts is sodium sulphate. Possibly some odour of a sulphurous nature is carried in the wind from the cave and acts as a cue for the elephants.

According to the wind direction, the sulphur smell might be detectable at a considerable distance from the entrance to the cave. The elephant might remember its association with salt. The putative sulphur odour cue would not explain how an elephant or the elephants found the needed sodium in the first place, which might have been by chance when the cave was only a small indentation under a lip of lava flow. It would not explain the precise navigation in pitch darkness to avoid the crevasses and reach the wall.

However, Redmond records recent experiments in which use of a global positioning system has allowed a herd of about 80 elephants to be tracked by the observers. These are the number remaining. They may move 15–20 km in a day, and are in the forest, but may make a clearly determined trek to the cave from several kilometres away. Sometimes they will stop along the way to feed. He says it is not possible to smell sulphur in the air. The elephants may pass known caves and go straight to Kitum cave ignoring the others. On one occasion when a BBC film crew, filming with Sir David Attenborough, had been installed in the cave with infra-red lights, the elephants who were monitored by the Mount Elgon Elephant Monitoring team (MEEM), created a pandemonium down in a bamboo forest, and then set off rapidly in the direction of Kitum Cave, through valleys and around ridges. The crew in the cave were reduced to two so as to least disturb the elephants. Only one young bull elephant, however, entered the cave, and mined the mineral rich rock, but he vocalized continually with a rumbling. Searching next morning showed numerous fresh elephant footprints and dung piles, both above and below the cave. It was clear that the elephants had gathered around the cave, but in the face of the smell of humans, had been unwilling to enter. The lone bull had entered (whether on his own volition or prompted by others as Redmond has wondered), and kept up a constant rumble to those outside. Whereas, none of the others entered the cave that night, a group of five entered the cave a few nights later with a calf. Subsequently, about 30 elephants entered and the BBC were able to film all this as the elephants became able to accept the presence of harmless observers, just as when Ian Redmond first went there. Ian Redmond notes that the MEEM team monitoring shows that the elephants have a good geographical knowledge. They don't just stumble by chance across Kitum or other caves they use. They know where the caves are and the best route to reach them—clear evidence, as he would see it, of intention.

It seems to me that the existence of an image in a conscious mind and execution of a plan based on past experience of what to do to get gratification when salt hunger begins to occupy the stream of consciousness is a more compelling hypothesis than random general appetitive behaviour. That is, the initial trek begins far from the cave site, and the animals follow learned jungle paths long before coming near enough to detect a 'certain something in the air'—any putative sulphurous or other smell.

A directly comparable situation, is where a grazing animal becomes gradually water depleted in hot conditions on grassland in the interior of a continent, and will trek many kilometres to a remembered water source. A common instance is on the cattle stations of the arid centre and north of Australia, where the only source of water is often from an artesian bore. The animals will trek out 10–15 miles to graze and then after 2–3 days return to the bore site at base to drink their fill. Trekking to a distant water source in the face of onset of dehydration would appear to be a striking example of the mental image of a goal beyond any immediate perception by sensory data—particularly if the water source is downwind. One can't ask the animal, but the acceptance of this has massive evolutionary consequences. In some ways this is very like accepting that animals can experience pain. As understood by the layperson or doctor, as Dr Grover Pitts (1994) has pointed out, pain means *conscious* suffering and is not experienced, for instance, by a surgical patient under anaesthesia. There is a philosophical abyss between the behaviourist definition of pain as withdrawal or flight in response to stimulation in any animal, vertebrate or invertebrate, and the anthropomorphic definition of pain as conscious suffering, which implies just that—consciousness of this particular type in animals.

A large body of natural history and observation of animal behaviour over centuries on several continents would ratify the dominance of salt (sodium chloride) need underlying mineral lick seeking behaviour of animals as recorded in the book The Hunger for Salt (Denton, 1983) referred to above. On the other hand, it is, I hope, of interest to mention here, in order to enlarge the background of the biology, that there are two metals other than sodium that may be relevant to the visit to the caves by the elephants. These are, phosphate and iron, and both, along with several other minerals, including manganese, magnesium, potassium, and calcium, are present in the fallen rock gouged out and eaten by the elephants. This raises other questions concerning instinctive determination of eating behaviour that may parallel salt appetite, and may be an additional motivation of the elephants.

The questions on phosphate appetite and iron intake involve fascinating aspects of behaviour of animals in the wild pertinent to our general theme. That is, they show intentional behaviour, at least, towards phosphate sources. This occurs when plasma phosphate concentration decreases. Laboratory experiments have revealed some of the processes (Blair-West *et al.*, 1992).

Part B

Experimental analysis

Chapter 6

Phylogeny, and the emergence of primary consciousness: Edelman's theory

The phylogenetic tree: first, to consider the phylogenetic tree as the framework of this account

Preceding chapters have described the intentional behaviour of animals in the wild, and laboratory experiments to explore their cognitive capacities. They have given evidence suggestive of consciousness in animals lower than the great apes. The material presented has not been exhaustive, but rather is illustrative. The reader should go to the in-depth, comprehensive accounts involving systematic analyses of particular criteria of conscious behaviour such as embodied in Donald Griffin's *Animal Minds* (1992). There is a rich collection of observation. Suffice to say, that, whereas consciousness in animals was once almost a taboo topic, most neurobiologists now accept it as a probable determinant of behaviour rather than an epiphenomenon, or that animals are simply automatons. Clearly the emergence of consciousness was the stellar event in animal evolution culminating in the dominance of the planetary environment and immediate regions of space by humans. The question emergent from the first part of the Chapter 4 dealing with animal behaviour would be, how far down the phylogenetic tree the possibility of consciousness would be accepted?

In recording the evidence at various levels of the phylogenetic tree, it is of high importance to take into account the disciplines of evolutionary analysis as set out by Hodos and Campbell (1990). That is, many present day species of vertebrates studied are not on the direct evolutionary line to *Homo sapiens*. As noted earlier, this applies to the teleost (bony) fishes, which are a separate line evolving in the ocean from an earlier ancestor that presumptively was ancestor to the early vertebrates that invaded the freshwater rivers. In the same vein, the birds are not on a direct line of evolution to humans. They represent a branch from the ancient reptiles, which were also the direct line to humans. Today the turtle represents the ancient reptilian common ancestor.

Hodos and Campbell (1990) and Butler and Hodos (1996) give a diagram (Fig. 6.1), which is representative of the *phylogenetic scale*—a figure they say is made up of imaginations and intuitions as there is no basis for it. Animals have a lower or higher place on the staircase depending on whether they are more complex. It carries the implication that the animals evolved in the indicated sequence, and those that appeared earlier in the sequence had lesser complexity. It reinforces an erroneous notion that animals have evolved along a single path leading to humans. In truth, the study of the fossil record indicates vertebrate evolution has proceeded along numerous independent paths. The evolutionary biologist has the model of a *phylogenetic tree* (Fig. 6.2). In this model there is no hierarchy. Birds are neither lower or higher than mammals but are merely on a different branch of the tree. The construction is multilinear. Geneological lines radiate out from a common origin. Different lineages evolve concurrently and independently of one another, and the tree is dependent on actual data and independent of complexity of biological function. Time is independent of the sequence so that different stages of evolution in different lineages can appear in the same epoch of time.

It would follow that consciousness as a property of the function of neural tissue may have evolved in differing ways in different irradiations during the course of development of living diversity. Again, in this regard, attention can

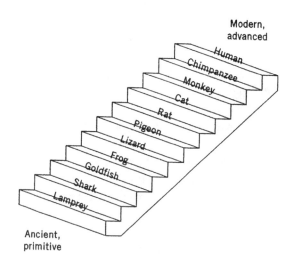

Figure 6.1 The so-called phylogenetic scale of vertebrates. The animals at the bottom are seen as being older and more primitive and less complex. The scale has no basis in fact. From A. Butler and W. Hodos *Comparative Vertebrate Anatomy*, Wiley-Liss, New York (Publishers), 1996. (With kind permission).

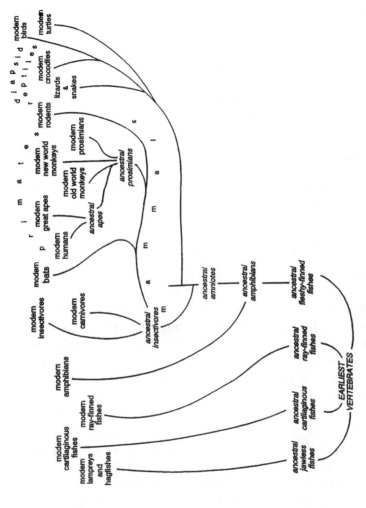

Figure 6.2 A phylogenetic tree of vertebrates in which there is no hierarchy. The animals at the bottom of the tree are phylogenetically older than those higher up. Birds are neither lower or higher than mammals, but are merely on a different branch of the tree. Evolutionary advancement is not indicated on this diagram. From A. Butler and W. Hodos *Comparative Vertebrate Anatomy*. Wiley-Liss, New York (Publishers), 1996. (With kind permission.)

be drawn to the remarkable differences in the mass of neurons of different species. Also there does not seem any simple relation of brain size and behavioural diversity. George Gabor Miklos (1998) of the Neuroscience Institute of La Jolla has stated that it is a widely held belief that more genes, more cell types, more neurons, more synapses, more axonal and dendritic arborization, and more glial cells give more morphological behavioural complexity. He thinks that there is much evidence contrary to such a belief. Of many examples, he cites the fact that 95% of nuclei (i.e. anatomically distinct concentrations of neurons in a particular locale) found in the rat brain are found in the human brain. The neuron numbers in miniature primates such as the pygmy marmoset (which is less than 10 cm in length and weighs only 168 gm, and has a brain volume of only 1.5 ml) must be near two orders of magnitude less than a chimpanzee, but the behavioural characteristics of these primates are broadly comparable.

Whereas the *scala naturae* (phylogenetic scale) suggests performance should vary by position on the staircase, the tree frees the behavioural scientist from predicting that always amphibians will perform more poorly than reptiles, that mammals will always surpass birds, that primates will always excel over other mammals. To illustrate, Hodos and Campbell (1990) go on to say that because birds follow a history quite independent from that of mammals, there is every reason to suppose that they may have evolved some capacities quite on their own that are superior to those of some mammals. They argue, in relation to statements whereby birds have been ranked lower than mammals, that in many ways birds have achieved the same grade as primates. For instance, birds are the only true bipedal species besides humans. Like primates, they have a complex social organization, a rich repertoire of vocal communication and they provide intensive and extended parental care. Birds use tools, they perform extremely well on tests of memory, and they have superb vision and visual perception. How many of the 'lower' mammals or higher non-primate mammals can boast the same abilities? Furthermore, they say, why should not alligators be ranked the same as birds as they provide parental care, establish territories, and defend them by vocalization and threat. It is known in the north of Australia that crocodiles exhibit good memory for places where food is likely. However, the experts in the Northern Territory of Australia in charge of parks do not ratify the story of crocodiles observing a person on the bank who repeatedly comes to the same place, and that the crocodile gradually edges closer each day, with only eyes visible, and finally makes a rush to capture the person.. Such behaviour, if substantiated, would suggest a goal and a plan, but presently the experts do not validate this folklore.

Descendant species have often undergone large modifications from their ancestral condition. The living descendants of ancestral lineages genetically should not be regarded as 'living fossils'. Does increase in complexity in relation to morphology or function necessarily mean progress or improvement? Hodos and Campbell (1990) cite the interesting case of the evolution of the vertebrate heart. They say one could construct a sequence of grades based on the number of chambers using the evolutionary scale, e.g. (1) fishes, (2) amphibians, and (3) amniotes (i.e. reptiles, birds, and mammals). At grade (1) we find a two-chambered heart, at grade (2) a three-chambered heart, and at grade (3) we have a four-chambered heart. Clearly there is an increase of complexity, and ostensibly progress. However, the data indicate that this is not an historical sequence. The division of the heart into four chambers appears to have occurred in the rhipidistian fishes, which were the fleshy finned ancestors of the amphibians (such as frogs). The three-chambered heart rather than representing a precursor of the four-chambered heart is *instead derived from the four-chambered heart*. This was a consequence of the amphibian reliance on the skin as an organ of respiration, in addition to the lungs. Because the amphibian skin is an efficient gas exchanger, the venous return to the heart from the body is well oxygenated. So there was no advantage in keeping blood from the body separate from the blood from the lungs.

The culminating consideration from this is that there are many lineages and diverse morphology emergent in the phylogenetic tree. Various lines of development evolve from the ancient forms, and these represent the continuity of the tree. It follows that there are many differing aspects of neural organization and brain function, and correspondingly, *it is conceivable that different forms of consciousness may have evolved.*

Edelman's theory on the emergence of primary consciousness

The development of the brain

In this section of the book I will acknowledge frequently my indebtedness to Gerald Edelman, who, with his collaborators, particularly Gulio Tononi, has in many ways been the leader of analytical debate on how primary consciousness emerged.

At the outset, I will detail some crucial elements in his views on the development of the brain, since his ideas on the emergence of the first dim awareness are set against that background. [Edelman has published a series of books, including: *Neural Darwinism, the Theory of Neuronal Group Selection* (1987); *The Remembered Present, a Biological Theory of Consciousness* (1989); *Bright Air, Brilliant Fire, on the Matter of the Mind* (1992); and *A Universe of Consciousness, How Matter becomes Imagination* (2000), the latter with Guilio Tononi as co-author.]

Charles Darwin's (1859) contribution, which Edelman terms 'the most ideologically significant of all grand scientific theories', centred on the idea that variation and diversity among individuals of a population provides the basis for competition and natural selection of the fittest. Thereupon they reproduce best. The process operates on the continual generation of diversity within a population. Edelman (1987) applies the same population notion to development of the brain and calls it 'Neural Darwinism'. Embodied in the idea is that,

1. During the early development of individuals, the forming of the anatomy of the brain is controlled by genetic forces. However, somatic selection determines the connectivity of synapses from the early stages of embryo development. Somatic means, *by events during the specific development of the individual.* It is what happens in the individual during its lifetime. The somatic events may be very short term over seconds, or last for very long periods.

In the period of ongoing development following birth, the intensity and frequency of events operating to contrive somatic selection of neural pathways will increase. During growth and development, individual neurons develop thousands of branching processes. In a given individual, extensive variability in the connection patterns will occur. An immense and diverse repertoire of connections results. Neurons also strengthen or weaken their synaptic connections according to the individual experience of electrical activity. Edelman's apt expression is 'Neurons that fire together, wire together'. That is, such neurons become closely connected.

---

2. Over the course of life, a process of synaptic selection occurs within neuronal populations as a result of behavioural experience. That is, the neuronal organization of the brain, its patterns of highly facilitated function subserved by synaptic selection, is sculptured by experience.

3. The third tenet of Edelman's concept is the process of 're-entry', which he delineates as quite different from feedback. Thus, feedback occurs in a single fixed loop of reciprocal connections. An error signal feeds back on the control system modifying its activity. However, he sees re-entry as contriving the synchronization of activity of neuronal groups in different brain maps. This binds them into circuits capable of a contemporaneous and coherent output. He sees it as the central mechanism by which coordination in space and time of diverse sensory and motor events takes place. An important example of the process would be in the instance of vision. Thus a property such as the colour of an object perceived in one modality of the brain would be linked with another involving motion.

Edelman (1987) terms his overall theory as NGST—Neuronal Group Selection Theory.

The parallel to antibody formation

There is a parallel, and Edelman draws it strongly, to the clonal selection theory of immunity proposed by an Australian Nobel Laureate, Sir MacFarlane Burnet. He proposed that an individual has the inherent ability to make a vast repertoire of antibody molecules, each of which has a different shape at its binding site. This is before the event of any encounter with a foreign (non-self) element—a bacterium or virus being classic instances. Thus, when the foreign molecule, which is part of a bacterium or virus is introduced into the body, it is confronted by a population of cells each with a different antibody on its surface. It binds to those cells that have antibodies with combining sites, more or less complementary to it. With a good fit, the cell carrying the antibody (the lymphocyte) is stimulated to divide repeatedly. Thus a clone, a progeny of cells, having antibodies of the same shape and specific capacity to bind is very rapidly built up. Thereupon, the lymphocyte population has been changed by selection. *This is called the clonal selection process, which distinguishes foreign molecules (non-self) from molecules of your own body (self).*

Edelman together with Rodney Porter, were responsible for analysis of the structure of an antibody. They received the Nobel Prize in 1972 for this work. It was shown that the polypeptide (protein) chains of an antibody involved constant regions and there were also variable regions that were different for each kind of molecule, and they comprised the binding site of an antigen (or foreign non-self molecules). This diversity in the variable region is generated somatically (that is within the individual's own lifetime) in the lymphocytes of each individual's body. As Edelman puts it, it involves a kind of jumbling within each lymphocyte of the genetic code specifying the variable antibody regions that may someday happen to bind to an antigen. Thus, the immune system is a relative recognition system. Moreover, the somatic diversity contrived in the variable regions may be such as to recognize a structure that never occurred before in the history of the planet.

In the broadest terms, the nub of Edelman's idea is that the function of the brain, including that termed the mind, arose in evolution as a result of two processes of selection: natural selection and somatic selection.

The emergence of primary consciousness

In describing Edelman's idea, I will stick closely to the language he uses to set it out.

He (1992) says that it is the evolutionary development of the ability to create a 'scene' that led to the emergence of primary consciousness. Primary consciousness he defines as the ability to construct an integrated mental scene in the present. It does not require language or a true sense of self. It is seen in animals with certain brain structures similar to our own. Higher order consciousness, epitomized in the human, presupposes the coexistence of primary consciousness, and involves a sense of self. This capacity for self-awareness has been described in many ways, such as Hughling Jackson's 'inward turning of consciousness', Isiaih Berlin's 'making the mind the subject and object of itself', or as conscious of being conscious.

Edelman suggests we experience primary consciousness as a 'picture' or 'mental image' of ongoing categorized events. Thus, the central element of the process is that *it is distance receptor generated*. By 'distance receptor' we are, in general, referring to the sensory capacities that detect events at a distance from the organisms integument, that is, outside itself—the eyes and the visual process, the ears and hearing, and the nose and smell.

The key element of the process of creating a 'scene' is perceptual categorization. Edelman says, *perceptual categorization* involves the process whereby the plethora of signals coming in from the external world at the same time, and they may not have any necessary causal or physical connection to one another, are carved up into signals which are useful for a particular species.

In relation to definition:

- Perception is defined as the discrimination of an object or event through one or more sensory modalities—separating them from the background inflow. Something is picked out.

- *Categorization* is a process whereby an individual may treat non-identical objects or events as equivalent. Thereupon, the individual generalizes on the basis of the category in relation to the action it will take. To this analysis, Edelman and Tononi (2000) have added the notion of 'concept', whereby different perceptual categorizations are combined to construct a 'universal'. This would reflect abstraction of some common features.

A cogent example of this theoretical view in relation to learning a concept on this basis is the experiments of Herrnstein and colleagues (1964, 1976)with pigeons, to which I referred briefly in Chapter 1. They are an extremely interesting and illustrative example. The hungry birds learnt to peck at a coloured slide picture that included a human, to achieve opening of a food hopper. In the experiment, when the pigeons were pecking more frequently at pictures with humans, a completely new set of pictures, positive and negative, were introduced and they pecked significantly more at pictures containing people (70–80% of the time). From these and other like experiments, Herrnstein, Loveland, and Cable (1976) proposed an animal readily forms a broad and complex concept. The birds had learned categories, and the concept was that this led to food. Herrnstein has also remarked that open-ended variability is the rule in nature rather than reproducibility or definiteness. Squirrels may learn where the acorns are but the acorns will vary in size, shape, and colour, and so will the oak trees. Mice may learn to be wary of houses and yards with cats in them even though the cats look different.

Edelman sees perceptual categorization along with control of movement, as the most fundamental process of the vertebrate nervous system.

It was proposed by Edelman and Tononi (2000) that at a time in evolutionary history, which roughly corresponded to the transition between reptiles and mammals on the one hand, and reptiles and birds on the other, a new anatomical connectivity emerged. It was critical.

> Primary consciousness emerged in evolution when, through the appearance of new circuits mediating re-entry, posterior areas of the brain that are involved in perceptual categorization were dynamically linked to anterior areas responsible for value based memory. This allowed the building of a remembered present—a scene that adaptively links immediate or imagined contingencies to that animal's previous history of value driven behaviour.

Thus the evolutionary derived re-entrant connectivity is implemented by several major systems of corticocortical fibres, which link the posterior cortex to the anterior parts. Presumptively, the posterior parts of the brain postulated to be involved would be largely those subserving vision. Also reciprocal connections linking the cortex and specific nuclei of the thalamus, including the reticular and intralaminar nuclei were basic to implementation. The thalamus is a large nuclear mass situated below the cortex. It is in the top part of the diencephalon, being situated between the midbrain and the cortex (Figs 9.1 and 11.2). Most inputs to the cortex are relayed through the synapses of the thalamus. Among other things, it is the great relay station of the sensory traffic from receptors in all parts of the body, as well as the upward flow of impulses from the brainstem and midbrain, including the reticular activating system. It is present in reptiles.

The intralaminar nuclei of the thalamus send diffuse projections to most areas of the cortex. All these thalamocortical structures and reciprocal connections acting via re-entry lead to the creation of a scene. (Edelman and Tononi 2000)

Now, coming back to Gerald Edelman's theory. When we consider a moving animal, parallel input from many different sensory modalities results in re-entrant correlations between complexes of perceptual categories related to objects and events. Edelman says that their *salience* is governed *by the activity of the animal's value systems, which involves memories of reward and punishment in the past.* The short-term memory, which is fundamental to primary consciousness reflects previous categorical and conceptual experiences. Thus, the ability to construct a conscious scene turns on the ability to construct within fractions of seconds a remembered present. He says, 'perceptual (phenomenal) experience arises from the correlation by a conceptual memory of a set of ongoing perceptual categorizations. Primary consciousness is a kind of "remembered" present.'

In his analysis, a predominant thought in Edelman's mind (Edelman 1992, Edelman and Tononi 2000) is that it is known fairly comprehensively which structures in the human brain are necessary and sufficient for consciousness. *The presence of such structures in the brain of an animal that shows immediate behaviour, which indicates exchange of signs, or of symbolic reference provides some anatomical justification for a working assumption that the animal is conscious. That is, the anatomical data are congruent with the behavioural data including the evidence of intention.*

Edelman, in the course of building a picture of the brain in his discourse in Daedalus (1998), the *Journal of the American Academy of Arts and Sciences*, suggests that an animal having primary consciousness alone can generate a 'mental image' or scene. This is based in part on immediate multimodal perceptual categorization in real time. It is determined by the succession of real events in the environment. He sees such an animal as having biological individuality but no concept of self. While it has a remembered present, it has no concept of the past or future.

This latter idea is perhaps debatable in that if it be conceded that the animal has a remembered present influenced by past reward and punishment (as stated above), the relevance of it would lie in a pertinent intention with, for example, a specific search determined to a greater or lesser degree by memory. However, as the issue before us is the very first emergence of primary consciousness, there is some element of puzzle as to how the process could be subserved by value category memory and 'the animal's own learned history' without this latter process having embodied a conscious experience.

Let us examine now Edelman's (1992) suggestion that the animal with primary consciousness has no concept of past or future. Such concepts emerged in evolution only when semantic capabilities emerged—perhaps earliest in the precursors of hominids. There seems little doubt that higher order consciousness flowered with linguistic capacity beginning in precursors of *Homo sapiens*. Speech allowed the description of feelings and the use of symbols. However, the possibility of intention seems to be implicit in some elements of Edelman's concept of 'the scene'. That is, it is inherent within the 'mental image' postulated. The survival advantage of the emergence of the ability to create a scene would turn to some extent on the action or intentionality implicit.

It could be argued that Edelman's proposal that primary consciousness arose with categorization of separate causally unconnected parts of the world (and these being correlated and bound into a scene) could represent a more advanced evolutionary stage than a primal emotion such as thirst, pain, or hunger. However, it is salient to Edelman's view that the optic tectum is a major anatomical feature in early living forms, as, for example, the lamprey, alligator, shark, and pigeon. It is the recipient of inflow from the optic nerves, and in many fishes it is larger than the cerebral hemispheres.

On this issue of early phylogenetic development, Ann Butler emphasizes that the paired eyes, and at least some parts of the hypothalamus and the epithalamus (the region of the pineal gland), appear to be present in the earliest craniate ancestors, which she terms cephalates. The craniate eyes arise embryologically by an initial midline outgrowth that then splits to form the bilateral pair of optic evaginations. Their relay to the tectum is a putative homologue of the cranial midbrain. She argues that the peripheral nervous system, including the olfactory system, and also the telencephalon were early additions, though later than the elaboration of the diencephalon and mesencephalon. That is, the paired eye system and hypothalamus anteceded the neural crest/neurogenic placode derived development of the peripheral nervous system. The telencephalon would have been tacked on as an additional, ultimate, rostral relay for these sensory pathways.

Furthermore, it is noteworthy in the octopus, the optic lobes contain a much greater mass of neurons than the verticalis lobe. This perhaps emphasizes the dominance of visual processing in this primitive creature. The octopus is, however, on a separate line of evolution from the lineage leading to the mammals.

As suggested earlier, *differing forms of consciousness, the apogee of the integrated functioning of neural aggregates, may have arisen in disparate ways on the phylogenetic tree.*

Edelman (1992) speculates that, given consciousness may be composed of phenomenal experiences, such as mental images, cold-blooded animals with primitive cortices would face severe restriction on primary consciousness because their value systems and value category memory lack a stable enough biochemical milieu in which to make linkages to a system that could sustain consciousness. So he says, 'Snakes are in (dubiously depending on the temperature) but lobsters are out. If further study bears out this surmise, consciousness is about 300 million years old'. *On the basis of contemporary comparative physiology, water drinking goes back this far, but the transition from what may have been reflex to that which may have been intentional could have involved the commencing colonization of land by the vertebrates. Hunger could be more primitive and go back much further phylogenetically.*

The synthesis of contemporary neuroanatomical and neurophysiological knowledge that Edelman has embodied in his theory of emergence of primary consciousness is a compelling, cogent, and imaginative exercise. It would seem likely to reflect fundamental features of the emergent functions of the brains of early vertebrates.

Recently, Edelman (2003) has elaborated his theory to embrace, to some extent, the idea I have proposed (1996), that the earliest element of consciousness may have involved the instincts dedicated to maintain homeostasis (i.e. the stability of the miliéu interiéur). This anneals with his central tenet that the 'creation of a scene' with perceptual categorization in the posterior parts of the brain is re-entrantly connected with frontal systems responsible for value category memory. He has now suggested that 'A ubiquitous set of inputs to the dynamic core is continually received from bodily and brain systems concerned with motor behaviour and homeostatic control. These inputs to the core are not only among the earliest but are also among the most persistent, and they provide a fundamental basis for subjectivity or the self-referential aspects of consciousness'.

Chapter 7

An interoceptor driven theory of origin of primary consciousness

An interoceptor theory

The theory I wish to propose is that primary consciousness arose from the primal or primordial emotions. Exemplars would be hunger for air, thirst, hunger, appetite for specific minerals such as salt hunger, sensations entrained by change of body core and body surface temperature, sexual excitation and orgasm and pain. The compelling desire to sleep after long deprivation would be a comparable instance of the invasion of consciousness with an internally generated primal emotion where little else can counter a desire that supersedes all other input. Similarly, the overfilling of the bladder and a compelling intention to void will give an imperious sensation akin to pain—or overdistension of the rectum can have a powerful distressing effect.

The theory is an alternative view to the Edelman theory that primary consciousness arose from the capacity to create a 'scene' with distance receptors as set out in Chapter 6. Here it is proposed that the evolutionary origin of consciousness came from primal emotions arising from chemical sensors and receptors, internal and some surface, which generated imperious sensation and an apt compelling intention, which signalled the immediate existence of the organism was threatened. Control of the basic vegetative systems involves genetically programmed neural organization that is centred in the ancient areas of the brain. The neural organization implicated is in the rhombencephalon (hindbrain), which includes the cerebellum, in the mesencephalon and the diencephalon, and with a central role for the reticular activating system and thalamic nuclei, as well as the phylogenetically ancient areas of the telencephalon—the forebrain. These latter are the allocortex (three cell layered) and transitional cortex (five cell layered), and include the anterior and posterior cingulate gyrus, the parahippocampus and the insula.

The limbic system, which includes these structures also has other areas, such as the dentate gyrus, and olfactory cortices including the piriform cortex, which are allocortex. Also part of the limbic system, which is the major cortical structure involved with primal emotion, is the collection of nuclei called the amygdala. The corticomedial amygdala is connected to the hypothalamus by way of a neural tract called the stria terminalis, and with the bed nucleus of the stria terminalis. The basolateral amygdala projects to the striatum (that is, the caudate nucleus, putamen, and globus pallidus), and is also widely interconnected with association areas of the isocortex—the six-layered areas.

The association areas of the cortex—the isocortex (frontal, parietal, occipital, and temporal) are six cell layered.

The midbrain regions involved within these structures control the elemental processes of arousal itself, and of sleep. As noted, the overwhelming sensation and desire which follows long deprivation of sleep, of itself, can be regarded as a primary emotion.

The limbic system

We will recount further on (Chapter 9) the result of neuroimaging of the onset, full development, and satiation of thirst. The heavy involvement of the limbic system of the cortex as well as regions lower in the human brain is described. It is apposite to give some background beforehand.

The limbic cortex was so named by Broca, a great French medical pioneer, because it was a rim on the medial surface of the brain surrounding the corpus callosum, which joins the two hemispheres of the brain. The cingulate gyrus, insula, and hippocampus together with their major brainstem connections are involved in a close functional integration. This functional integration was first elaborated by Papez (1937), a neuroanatomist in New York.

As LeDoux of New York has summarized it, Papez proposed the genesis of emotion resided in an anatomical circle. That is, sensory inputs into the brain are split in the thalamus into what amounts to a stream of thought and a stream of feeling. The streams of thought are transmitted via the thalamus to the lateral areas of the neocortex where they are processed to perception, thoughts and memories. The stream of feeling was relayed from the thalamus to the hypothalamus—to the mammillary bodies there. These relay them on to the cortex. Specifically this is to the old cortex, the cingulate, which relays the signals on to the hippocampus and back to the hypothalamus. Within the circuit, it was also envisaged that the higher areas, which had processed the stream of thought, might also give rise to emotion by themselves relaying on to the cingulate.

Some later workers in the anatomical and physiological field—Brodal and LeDoux himself, and Blessing of Australia—have doubted the value of the concept of the limbic system. They stress the complexity of hypothalamic connections with the cortex. Notwithstanding, the use of the term 'limbic system' does serve to identify a group of functionally related structures. Experiments have shown them to underpin a variety of emotional and vegetative functions. The areas embraced by the term are evolutionary ancient brain regions. The parahippocampus, amygdala, and thalamus are present in reptiles and amphibians. The five-layered cortex of the cingulate region appears in the earliest mammals. However, views differ regarding the phylogeny of these limbic areas. Butler and Hodos (1996) state that the current evidence indicates that the limbic system evolved long before the advent of any amniote vertebrates (i.e. before the mammals, and diapsid reptiles such as lizards, snakes, and crocodiles). Amniotes have a membrane and amniotic fluid surrounding the embryo. Diapsid means the skull has two temporal openings and two arches of bone. So the limbic system came long before the mammals.

Thus, as we will show, the heavy involvement of limbic areas in thirst is consistent with thirst being a primitive vegetative function with much of its circuitry emergent early in vertebrate evolution. Indeed, in our neuroimaging of thirst, it was found that 14 regions of the Papez circuit were highly significantly activated. Also there were nine highly significant deactivations. It possibly reflects that the cingulate cortex is the only portion of the telencephalic cortex with strong hypothalamic connections.

Grossman (1980) of Texas writing on the emergence of consciousness says that,

> whereas . . . the anterior thalamic, and also mesencephalic and pontine brainstem are necessary for consciousness they are probably not sufficient. Interaction of these rather small masses of neurons with, at least, a certain volume of limbic or neocortex must occur. The thalamic and brainstem areas may function as organizers of cortical activity and probably must themselves be included in cortical-subcortical-cortical circuits for consciousness to occur.

Consistent with this view, it could be that the evolutionary process whereby the primitive hindbrain grew rostrally (frontwards) involved both anatomical elaboration and functional emergence of specialized sections that were necessary for the emergence of consciousness. Then cellular architecture of the cortex developed. The key corticothalamic connections, and the direct connections of the thalamus to hypothalamus, mesencephalon, medulla, and the motor regions of the striate complex evolved. One could speculate that *this allowed the complex genetic reflex mechanisms of the hypothalamus, midbrain, and hindbrain, which had determined vegetative behaviour to now be modified spectacularly by thalamic and cortical development resulting in emergent conscious awareness embodying intention and with the subjectivity inherent. The creature could then begin to exercise options.*

Genetically programmed neural connections

Estimates of up to a hundred billion neurons have been given for the number of neurons in the brain. A neuron may have up to ten thousand dendrites or processes capable of forming connections with other nerve cells. It follows that the number of possible combinations of connections that could develop between neurons is of cosmic dimensions. It was initially thought that the number of genes in the human genome was of the order of a hundred thousand but sequencing studies have indicated that the number is nearer thirty thousand, with the largest proportion being believed to be expressed in the brain. Such a number could include genes involved in the coding of neural networks and the sensors subserving a diversity of innate behaviour patterns. The genetic coding of facility of connection underlying particular neural networks could underpin the genetic propensity to learn special behaviours that involve complexity of action.

Presumptively such 'hard wired' or genetically programmed neural connections are the basis of the instincts. It is clear that such hard wiring may be strongly conserved in ascent of the phylogenetic tree because of the very high survival value of specific instincts. Thus, drinking is elicited in response to an increase of the salt concentration of the blood by about 2%, and this holds in all mammals, including humans. A similar effect is achieved by injection into the brain of the peptide hormone angiotensin II. This hormone is a major neurotransmitter in the neural systems, which subserve the evocation of thirst and the desire to drink in mammals. The evocation of drinking behaviours by these manoeuvres goes, however, very much lower in the phylogenetic tree. Bony fish may be made to drink by raising the salt concentration of the blood, and reptiles such as iguanas respond to injection of angiotensin into the brain by drinking.

Whereas there are many instincts, such as thirst and drinking—which are based on genetically programmed neural organization, it is obvious from the quantitative consideration at the outset of this section (i.e. the cosmic number of connections feasible) that the genetically determined hard wiring could not account for all the vast capacities for learning and adaptation manifest in the function of the nervous system of animals. A totally different concept is necessary in the approach to the functional organization of the brain. Such a concept is enunciated in Gerald Edelman's theory of Group Neuronal Selection, which was described earlier.

Instincts

There is a very great diversity of instincts. There are instinctive behaviours that are elements of the vegetative systems of the body. They are directed to the maintenance of the chemical and physical constancy of the internal environment. Such dominant functions are controlled by sensors within the body, which detect deviation from normal. They include the hunger for air determined by increase of the carbon dioxide of the blood (in higher animals decreased oxygen content of the blood is a much weaker stimulus to air hunger). There is thirst, and also there is hunger for food. This latter is caused, among other factors, by a reduction of glucose concentration in blood. Hunger for salt (sodium) is a very powerful instinct, and it is caused by change of sodium concentration of the blood in the herbivorous species and by action in the brain of angiotensin and the salt-retaining hormone aldosterone in other species. Hunger for other metallic ions, such as calcium or phosphorus is caused also by reduction of blood level of these ions, or by hormonal changes set in motion by the depletion of body stores. Also, with the reproductive process where increased body need of sodium and calcium arise, hormones stimulate the brain receptors, which determine the specific appetites for sodium and calcium salts. To this list could be added the behavioural sequelae caused by rise or decrease in the temperature of blood going to brain, which is detected by sensors. That is, brain sensors as distinct from detectors of skin temperature change. These brain sensors can cause involuntary actions, such as shivering and panting. Apart from this they can invoke behaviours that contrive amelioration of the temperature effects such as vigorous nest building in the cold as beautifully shown by Curt Richter (1976) of Johns Hopkins University.

A plethora of instinctive sexual behaviours are involved in the reproductive processes. They are choreographed by changes in the concentration of sex hormones in the blood, often on a cyclic basis. These blood changes entrain chemical changes within brain cells which are specific. The cells have special receptors for the hormones and they are wired to other brain cells to initiate motor mechanisms of sexual behaviour. This could be anything from dancing in birds, to lordosis in the female rat in response to physical pressure of the male. Many behaviours are related also to a territorial competition with conspecifics, and then aggression results. As such, the behaviours reflect, *inter alia*, a situational perception again often activated by hormone changes in the blood.

Instinct and emotion

Without continuing such a catalogue of instincts, the overview I would like to suggest is the statement of William James (1890) noted in the Introduction. 'In speaking of the instincts it has been impossible to keep them separate from the emotional excitements which go with them.' Further, 'Instinctive reactions and emotional expressions thus shade imperceptibility into each other. Every object which excites an instinct excites an emotion as well.'

A similar viewpoint was stated by W. McDougall (1923) in '*An Outline of Psychology*'—namely, that humans had just as many instincts as he had qualitatively distinguishable emotions. Verwey, a great student of the behaviour of the grey heron wrote 'where reflexes and instincts can be distinguished from each other at all, there the reflex is functioning mechanically, while instinctive activities are accompanied by subjective phenomena' (translated from German by Konrad Lorenz, 1950).

The *Oxford Dictionary* in its definition of emotion delineates emotions arising from bodily states as well as those arising in other ways.

The thesis being followed in this book centres on the primal emotions arising from the instinctive programmes of the vegetative systems. Our viewpoint is that the interoceptor engineered imperious sensation has an inherent compulsive intention whether it be to gasp for air, to drink, to eat, to pass water, or escape a pain if possible. James (1890) appears to be saying this in his linking of an emotion with an instinctive reaction, the two shading imperceptibly into each other.

Whereas what James (1890) was saying is particularly apposite to the vegetative systems, he was, in fact, particularly directed towards human instincts dependent on situational perception. That is, instincts determined by distance receptor inflow. He noted their full physiological impact. '...objects of rage, love, fear etc., not only prompt a man to outward deeds but provoke characteristic alterations in his attitude and visage and affect his breathing, circulation and other organic functions in specific ways.'

James' focus on the visceral reactions led him with Lange to propose a theory of emotion, which suggested that the visual perception of a situation set in train visceral reactions, and it was the brain's perception of these evoked bodily changes that constituted the emotion. Whereas such visceral reactions do feed back and contribute to the complexities of the conscious state, it is now accepted that the emotional state is primarily generated in the brain.

The primitive motor system, the sense of self and the body image

Given what I proposed above—that the primal emotions of the vegetative systems are the beginning of consciousness—it is important to recount that Jaak Panksepp (1998) proposes a different idea on origin. Like the primal emotion theory, it also places the evolutionary genesis of consciousness in the brainstem, in contrast to the largely exteroceptor visual function as proposed by Edelman (1992, 1998) (Chapter 6). However, it generally bases the origins with the primordial motor systems in this region of the brain.

Jaak Panksepp (1998) puts considerable emphasis on the data from split brain studies, which would seem to affirm that the essential centre of existence is subcortical. Despite instances of the sinister left hand opposing the action of the right as recounted by Sperry (1974), the split brain individual functions in the main as a co-ordinated individual. It requires special experiments to demonstrate the profound differences in perceptual awareness of the hemispheres. In parallel, it is also true that, with massive damage of portions of the human cortical mantle by a stroke, the internally sustained neural representation of the person as a coherent individual remains intact. That is, this subcortical region is the centre of self, which he says is the basis of animals experiencing themselves as active, feeling creatures in the world.

In an imaginative analysis of this proposal of primitive attentional and intentional forces, he places the emphasis on the primordial motor processes within the brainstem. He says '. . . the SELF (Simple Ego Life Form) first arises during early development from a coherently organized motor process in the midbrain, even though it surely comes to be represented in widely distributed ways through higher regions of the brain as a function of neural and psychological maturation.' Thus, the primordial self-schema was laid out first in stable motor co-ordinates within the brainstem—in the periventricular and surrounding areas of the midbrain and diencephalon, which are richly connected with higher limbic and paleocortical zones. *He sees these primal motor areas as the most likely source of the primitive neural mechanisms, which generate affective states of consciousness.* The primordial circuits generate a fundamental sense of 'self' within the brain, which allows animals to develop into the intentional and volitional creatures that they are.

Panksepp (1998) states it is easy to overlook this motor foundation of consciousness when we are continually entranced by the protean forms of sensory—perceptual awareness.

This idea of Panksepp of a motor basis of emergence of consciousness has a coherence—an empathy—with the earlier general reflection of Homer Smith (1959) (Chapter 3). This was that consciousness first emerged when animals developed the capacity to go from here to there in search of food. Indeed, there was no requirement for awareness of environment or self in the individual until it develops the physical ability to move and the neuromuscular system to do it.

Panksepp sees the archaic self-representation network as controlling motor tone and basic orientating responses. Also its intrinsic rhythms can be varied by a wide range of regulatory inputs. It is highly interactive with all the emotional circuitry. Overall, feelings may take effect when '. . . endogenous sensory and emotional systems within the brain that receive direct inputs from the outside world as well as the neurodynamics of the SELF begin to reverberate with each other's changing neuronal firing rhythms'.

Panksepp argues further that this primitive self-representation, supporting affective states, becomes the psychic scaffolding for all other forms of consciousness. Thus, primary process consciousness will not be seen simply as awareness of external events in the world but as an ineffable feeling of experiencing oneself as an active agent in the perceived events of the world. This point was emphasized by J.Z. Young (1986) in drawing attention to the views of the Viennese philosopher Brentano, as being pertinent to the notion of intention. Brentano noted that conscious intention may involve a distinction between the creature's own thoughts, and the sensory information coming from the outside. In relation to the locus of the SELF Panksepp (1998) says, whereas this is uncertain, the deep cerebellar nuclei receive a great deal of primitive sensory and emotional information, and control body movements, especially those directed by sensory feedback. The centromedial areas of the midbrain, including the deep layers of the colliculi and periventricular gray do the same. As removal of the cerebellum does not impair consciousness, the centromedial zone of the midbrain is, in Panksepp's eyes, the epicentre of the SELF.

Considering this hypothesis of Panksepp's, which is, in effect, dealing with the first dawning of consciousness, there is, I suppose relative to the one I have put forward in this chapter and elsewhere, the issue of what comes first. In a way, with the hypothesis I have raised for consideration, the primal or primordial emotion as the generative phenomenon carries an amalgam of the imperious sensation and the compelling intention as in the definition proposed in Chapter 12. The implication is that the former is generally causal of the latter. This is not to gainsay that a large portfolio of reflex mechanisms in the brainstem at early stages of phylogeny subserve response to disturbance of the miliéu interiéur, or to external stimuli. However, no conscious sensation is involved in the reflex motor responses even if complex. Possibly the drinking response of fish in salt water is entirely reflex without any conscious component. The essential idea advanced in the primordial emotion theory was that it was at a certain stage of evolution involving rostral (forward) growth of the brain that consciousness first entered the biological process, and motor activity became intentional. That is, considering the thirst process again, the primal subjective awareness that the body was desiccating was causal of both the intention and motor events of seeking of water. This happened very early in the migration of animals out of the rivers and swamps to free living existence on dry land.

This general issue of cause and effect is pertinent to the debate. Logically, the proposition would be that the cause precedes the effect in time, the effect is not present without the cause, and there is a commensurate relation between cause and effect (the bigger the stimulus the greater the response). It is particularly interesting that John Searle (1989) has used thirst as a major illustration of the issue of intentional causation in his 1984 Reith Lectures for the BBC, and in his book *Intentionality* (1983). Whereas I would note that drinking may occur without thirst, as is evidently the case with human socially conditioned drinking of beverages often at ritually determined times of day, it is true in animals and often in humans that drinking is determined by thirst. Thirst arises from nerve firings in the hypothalamus caused by change of blood composition as a consequence of desiccation. Searle states that to be thirsty is to have among other things the desire to drink; thirst therefore is an intentional state. It has content and its content determines under which conditions it is satisfied, and it has all the rest of the features common to intentional states.

Intentional states cause things to happen by way of intentional causation to bring about a match—that is to bring about a state of affairs they represent, their own conditions of satisfaction. As Searle puts it, actions characteristically consist of two components, a mental component and a physical component. The mental component is an intention and is about something. If successful the mental component causes the physical component 'This form of causation I call intentional causation, and it is an intention to do something'. Consonant with what I have noted above about differing causes of drinking, Searle's formal analysis points out, whereas there is the statement that he took a drink because he was thirsty, and the counterfactual statement that he didn't take a drink because he was not thirsty, there is not necessarily any universal law involved. The second time around when thirsty, he may not have taken a drink. It was up to him.

Notwithstanding the delineation of the complexity of this basic physiological regulation in relation to causation as embodied in Searle's discussion, a key viewpoint is that 'the mental energy that is identified as powering action is an energy that works by intentional causation'.

In my eyes it is plausible phylogenetically that the emergence of the consciousness of sensory inflow came before the conscious employment of motor systems to bring about conditions of satisfaction of the causative mental state. Basically, the awareness of sensory inflow caused the selection pressure that favoured the portfolio of complex reflex motor mechanisms of the mid- and hindbrain to evolve also towards conscious, and, thus, volitional control.

What I am saying on this crucial point would appear to be in accord with some reflections of William James (1890) on the consciousness of self. Referring to the stream of consciousness he says,

> if the stream as a whole is identified with the Self far more than any outward thing, a certain portion of the stream abstracted from the rest is so identified in an altogether peculiar degree, and is felt by all men as a sort of innermost centre within the circle of sanctuary within the citadel, constituted by subjective life as a whole.

He asks 'What is this self of all other selves?' and suggests common viewpoint would call it the active element in all consciousness ... 'it is that within us to which the pleasant and painful speak. It is what welcomes or rejects. It presides over the perception of sensations and, by giving or withholding its assent, it influences the movements they tend to arouse. It is the source of effort and attention, and the place from which appear to emanate the feats of the will.'

Panksepp (1998), however, has suggested that a level of motor coherence had to exist before there would be utility for sensory guidance. *However, this would not rule out the alternative that the motor coherence was a co-ordinated reflex system—non-conscious—upon which the dawning consciousness of sensation was phylogenetically imposed.*

Panksepp's idea that the core of the SELF is situated in the ancient circuits of the midbrain is strongly supported, as he points out, by the fact that the extended ascending reticular activating system, including the thalamic reticular nuclei, control the essential waking and attentional functions of the brain. Overall, whether or not it was the primordial interoceptor driven emotional sensation or the motor activity so evoked, which was the prime mover of origin of consciousness, the reality is that they are deeply entwined. Both ideas place the genesis or epicentre of consciousness in the brainstem. These phylogenetically ancient parts are the console of the organ, as Jean-Pierre Changeux (1985) puts it, and they play the cortical mantle. The argument that they are the prime core of SELF is well supported by the fact cited that large cortical lesions as a result of stroke can eliminate a variety of specific abilities such as speech, or even awareness of a side of the body without destroying the patient's sense of being a coherent individual. However, if the core area in the periventricular gray and the ascending reticular activating system and pontine nuclei is damaged, consciousness is lost.

In this regard, it is perhaps cogent that in the horrendous 'locked in' syndrome, a lesion in the anterior pontine area destroys all motor activity in the body except a capacity to move the eyes vertically. The patient remains fully conscious despite virtually complete motor loss. On the other hand, lesion in the posterior pontine area with destruction of ascending sensory pathways and reticular activating cells results in coma.

We will discuss further aspects of emotions in the context of a general overview in Chapter 12. We will now look at the physiological basis of thirst and what is revealed by imaging the brain during experience of the primal emotion of thirst, and its satiation by drinking.

Chapter 8

The physiology of the primordial emotion of thirst

The issues to be discussed

This chapter precedes the pivotal Chapter 9, which records what happens in the neuroimages of the brain when the primal emotion of thirst invades the stream of consciousness. Here, the reader can learn of the physical changes in the body that produce thirst, and the organization that subserves it at different levels of evolutionary development. The account emphasizes that water drinking is an ancient behaviour. Further, the fact that 'dryness of the mouth' was once incorrectly believed to be the prime cause of thirst is described. Of great importance in this chapter, we describe how satiation of thirst by drinking water causes immediate precipitate disappearance of thirst. This is even though the chemical changes in the body that caused thirst in the first place are unchanged until water is absorbed from the gut much later. This trick of immediate gratification has very high survival value for animals. Study of it may provide a royal road for seeing, with neuroimaging and electrophysiological studies, which activations in the brain subserve the actual consciousness of thirst and disappear, and which parts react to chemical changes in the body and persist.

Section A—the mechanisms producing thirst

Much of this chapter is marked to indicate that the lay reader might pass it without loss of the thread.

Rullier in 1821 in the *Dictionaire des Sciences Medicales par un Societé de Medicins et Chirurgiens*, said of thirst '. . . *le sentiment le plus vif et les plus imperieux de la vie.*'

In light of the idea that phylogenetically ancient areas of the brain would subserve the primal emotions, it seemed of crucial importance to neuroimage what happens in the brain when the powerful primal emotion of thirst is evoked. Classical neurophysiological studies—electrical stimulation and recording of brain activity, study of effect of lesions and molecular biological techniques have aimed to reveal which neurons are activated. The methods have shown clearly that some brainstem loci play a major part in thirst.

However, it was not known in the genesis of thirst which cortical areas link up with the crucial brainstem areas such as the anterior wall of the third ventricle in the hypothalamus. Cortical areas might be presumed to be essential because it is most unlikely that the consciousness of thirst would arise only from the small population of cells in the front wall of the third ventricle. This is notwithstanding that this third ventricle region is essential to thirst and drinking behaviour. It is likely to be one of the jointly sufficient and severally necessary factors in determining thirst.

Before recounting results from brain imaging of thirst it is desirable to review some general physiological questions that are relevant.

1. How is a sense of thirst generated? What is the change in the physical state of the body which causes it?
2. Where is that change in the physical state of the body detected?
3. When did the thirst system first develop in the course of evolution of animal life?
4. How did the medical ideas on thirst develop and did they give insight into fundamental aspects of that complex phenomenon?

Change of osmotic pressure and sodium concentration

The terms 'osmotic pressure', and 'change of osmotic pressure' are used in the analysis of changes in body fluids. At its simplest, osmosis is the movement of water between two solutions with different concentrations of dissolved substances such as salts or sugars when the solutions are separated by a semipermeable membrane. This is when they are separated by a membrane such as a membrane of a living cell, which is permeable to water but impermeable to most solutes (dissolved substances). In such a case, water will tend to move from the compartment with a lesser concentration of solute to the one with the higher concentration of solute until the concentrations become equal. The osmotic pressure is the pressure required to stop this movement. That is, the pressure necessary to counteract the movement of water is the difference of osmotic pressure between the two solutions.

In the case of the cells of the animal body, the main metallic element (cation) is potassium, and there are also small amounts of magnesium, calcium, sodium, and other metallic ions. These positive metallic ions are balanced in terms of electrical charge by negative ions (anions), such as chloride, phosphate, bicarbonate, and organic molecules. The cell membrane is relatively impermeable to all these ions but is permeable to water. Surrounding the cells of the body there is the circulating miliéu interiéur, or extracellular fluid, which includes the plasma of the blood. The main metallic ion (cation) of the miliéu interiéur is sodium, and there are also small amounts of potassium, calcium, and magnesium. The electrically balancing amount of the negative ions (anions) is made up of chloride, bicarbonate, phosphate, and other components. If there is loss of fluid from the extracellular compartment as a result of secretions not being reabsorbed, this fluid may often contain a considerable amount of water in excess of electrolytes relative to the relation of the two in the extracellular compartment. This will happen, for example, with sweating (sweat contains 40–50 millimoles of sodium per litre compared with 150 millimoles per litre in the extracellular fluid). At the extreme, the same thing happens as a result of expiration of water from the lung with breathing.

In the absence of replacement of water, loss of water from the extracellular compartment causes the concentration of sodium, and, thus, the overall osmotic pressure of the extracellular compartment to rise. This will withdraw water from the cells of the body. *That is, cellular dehydration occurs.* The same effect is achieved by the infusion into the bloodstream of a saline solution that is more concentrated than the normal concentration of sodium in the blood.

However, there is a difference. With the loss of fluid from the body by sweating and respiratory expiration, the volume of the blood plasma and extracellular fluid also decreases. However, in the case of the infusion of concentrated salt, it will increase. This has some implications because, apart from change of sodium concentration, reduction of volume of blood and circulating extracellular fluid can itself stimulate thirst. However, the essential fact is that in either case, the sodium concentration of the extracellular fluid (it is by far and away the major component of dissolved substances) and the osmotic pressure both rise. This rise in sodium and osmotic pressure will overrule any effect the expansion of volume of extracellular fluid caused by infusion of fluid would have in blunting thirst.

The location of the sensors of change of osmotic pressure

Now in relation to dehydration of cells of the body, specific cells in the brain that participate in this change are situated on the front wall of the third ventricle in the hypothalamus (Figs 9.1(a) and 9.6). There are 'wired up' so that they act as sensors of this general change. All cells of the body would shrink somewhat as a result of the rise of salt concentration of the extracellular fluid, but the sensors are 'wired' to send out impulses. This they do to other areas of the brain, which are in some way, as yet mysterious, involved in the processes of contriving the emergence of the consciousness of thirst. Surgical destruction of this area on the front wall of the third ventricle of the brain causes loss of thirst. The animal or human loses partially or entirely the desire to drink despite a very high salt concentration of the blood.

The operation of the sensing system in the third ventricle region is actually more complex. That is, a rise in osmotic pressure of the blood and tissue fluids will stimulate thirst but also cause the release of a hormone, vasopressin, from the pituitary gland situated at the base of the brain. This hormone acts to cause the kidney to retain water. At a regulatory level this complements thirst. However, whereas vasopressin helps offset the consequences of water loss, it is obvious that it is only the thirst process and resulting water intake that can restore the physiological state to normal.

As well as sensors responsive to osmotic pressure, there are other elements within the region of the third ventricle that are specifically responsive to the concentration of sodium itself. When a rise in sodium concentration of the cerebrospinal fluid occurs, which will usually be the case when a rise of osmotic pressure of blood occurs, this effect will concurrently stimulate these special sensors responsive specifically to change of sodium concentration, and it will cause thirst. However, the operating role of these sensors, which specifically react to sodium concentration becomes evident with an experimental procedure. That is, the sodium concentration of the brain extracellular fluid can be reduced by an infusion of saline with a lower sodium concentration than normal into the ventricles of the brain. If this is done at the same time that the osmotic pressure of the blood and tissue fluids (extracellular fluid) of the body rises, then characteristic thirst inducing effect of the rise of osmotic pressure of the body tissue fluid is reduced or stopped. This has been found by Andersson and Olsson of Stockholm, and by our group at the Howard Florey Institute. Further, at the Howard Florey Institute in Melbourne, it has been shown that not only will decrease of sodium concentration in brain fluids decrease thirst, but it will also stimulate a hunger for salt (Denton 1983). This is a most apt response if the salt concentration of the miliéu interiéur is falling. This would happen with protracted loss of sodium salts from the body, associated with continuation of water drinking stimulated by a reduction of the volume of circulating extracellular fluid.

Evolution of thirst and drinking behaviour

The emergence of drinking behaviour during the course of evolution has been extensively analysed by James Fitzsimons of the Department of Physiology at University of Cambridge. He has been a world leader in this field, and his book on thirst is a classic (1979). He, together with Bengt Andersson and Kerstin Olsson of Uppsala and Stockholm Universities in Sweden, Michael McKinley of the Howard Florey Institute in Melbourne, Ed Stricker of Pittsburg, Kim Johnson of Iowa, and others, including the earlier workers, Wolf and Adolph in the USA, have pioneered this field.

Overall, and particularly the comparative studies of Fitzsimons (1979) and Japanese workers including Kobayashi and Hirano, have indicated that drinking behaviour—the seeking of water—emerged very early in the evolution of vertebrates in response to the environmental selection pressures involved. This has implications in the phylogeny of consciousness.

Aquatic animals

As James Fitzsimons (1979) has set out in his book, animals that live in water require less water than those that live on dry land because there are no thermoregulatory or respiratory water losses, and thus their water needs are relatively constant. Animals living in freshwater from protozoa upwards are hypertonic (that is, they have higher osmotic pressure) than their surrounding milieu. The major problem presenting for them is to deal with the osmotically determined inflow of water, and any loss of electrolytes that occurs from their skin. With ascent of the phylogenetic tree, the methods of getting rid of water range from the contractile vacuole in creatures such as the amoeba to the spectacular evolutionary jump represented by the emergence of the glomerulotubular kidney as described in Chapter 5.

Animals in seawater have an opposite problem. Confining the discussion to the marine animals with backbone, the tissue fluids and cells are hypotonic relative to the concentration of electrolytes in seawater. That is, they have lower osmotic pressure than the surrounding sea. Therefore, they lose water by osmosis and gain electrolytes by diffusion through exposed membranes and also in the course of eating. The strategy of coping with this differs with different species. Considering the bony fishes of the sea, they drink the seawater that surrounds them, and then dispose of excess sodium chloride by actively secreting it from the gills. They get rid of magnesium and sulphate in their urine. There is a net gain of the water they need. The migratory bony fish such as salmon and eel are very interesting because in fresh water they don't drink and excrete copious urine, whereas in seawater they drink, excrete salt from their gills, and the rate of glomerular filtration in their kidneys falls so that they produce very little urine. The amphibia had begun to colonize the land in the late Devonian period about 300 000 000 years ago, and spent part of the time in water and part on dry land. Their kidneys adapted to this situation by excreting much urine when in the water, but ceased to do so when on dry land. A mark of adaption of the amphibian is the capacity to take up water through its skin. It is noteworthy that many amphibia do not show water seeking behaviour when dehydrated.

Reptiles and birds

Reptiles are the first terrestrial vertebrates. They emerge in the Upper Carboniferous and Permian periods, about 200 000 000 years ago, and have colonized diverse ecosystems of the earth. Their evolutionary trick of enclosing their offspring in membranes impermeable to water was a great advantage. They weren't exposed to predators as would have been the case if the young had developed in ponds or streams. The closed egg contains its own water supply, and is suitable for the developing embryo.

Another feature of their adaption to dry land was the fact that they developed the capacity to excrete the products of nitrogen metabolism as uric acid rather than the basic ammonia or the water soluble urea. Water was reabsorbed from the urine in the renal tubules and cloaca, and uric acid, which is not very soluble precipitated in the cloaca to form a semi-solid mixture of urine and faeces. This will be familiar to all in the deposits of birds on one's car. That is, this uricotelism, as it is called, is a feature of reptiles and birds. It is also important in the development of embryo within the closed egg and with a limited water supply.
Other reptiles, such as the turtles help to control their osmotic balance by having nasal glands that secrete what appear to be tears but are solutions of sodium chloride more concentrated than blood. This allows a net gain of water. Marine birds also do this.

As Fitzsimons (1979) pointed out, many reptiles also drink when allowed water after a period of water deprivation. The drinking of water in response to water deprivation by an animal on dry land requires a sequence of motivated behaviours. They first seek water and then ingest it in appropriate amounts. This is a much more complicated behaviour pattern than simply opening the mouth and swallowing water as is the case with fish. It is conceivable that this may delineate a stage at which some conscious processes developed.

With birds, new components of the kidney tubules first emerged. This allows the production of a urine more concentrated than the circulating milieu with relative water saving. This mechanism combined with the excretion of nitrogen end products as uric acid, together with nasal salt glands in marine birds and also in some terrestrial species, has helped them take advantage of salty water for their supply of water. Most birds do drink with the exception of some that get their water supply from their food.

Migration

As mentioned earlier, James Fitzsimons has stated, 'It is a moot point whether or not fish experience thirst, a conscious sensation leading to motivated drinking behaviour.' He noted that when an eel is transferred to fresh water it stops drinking but it will drink again if hypertonic sodium chloride is infused intravenously or it is bled, or, angiotensin is injected into it. Overall, it appears the immediate onset or cessation of drinking when euryhaline (broad adaptability to saline content of the environment) fish move between freshwater and seawater seems to depend on chloride sensitive receptors on the surface of the body (palatal organ, lateral line organ, and the olfactory system) and not on the dehydrating effect of seawater. That is, the receptors anticipate effects.

It would appear that the drinking behaviour of fish could be reflexly determined by external sensors, as well as sensors within the body in response to chemical change. The latter may also account for cessation of the drinking process. The essential point is that water whether fresh or salt surrounds the creature and response can occur without the need of other behaviour. Fitzsimons noted that eels continue to drink after removal of their forebrain and midbrain. The hypothalamus, therefore, appears to have little to do with the control of drinking. As water is everywhere, the neural mechanisms necessary to ensure intake could be much simpler than the terrestrial creature where the repertoire of behaviour of seeking and ingesting water is much more complicated. Then, increased encephalization (involvement of forward areas of the brain) becomes necessary.

As we noted earlier, amphibia can respond like freshwater fish. However, when they utilize lungs on land they will lose water but they can repair this by absorbing water through the skin. The evidence is against intake being a behaviourally controlled process as one might have been expected. A dehydrated frog in a laboratory near a pool of water does not show any water seeking behaviour. It can die of lack of water though only a few centimetres from the pool.

This was shown by Professor Adolph (1943). However, should it stumble on water through movement on land it stays there. Thus it may react to the need for and a benefit derived from water according to Adolph. It seems that the additional mechanism of locating water in order to absorb it is not within the range of the nervous system in this animal, which is close to being a fish.

Reptiles, which are the first truly terrestrial vertebrates, made the vital adaptation in being able to engage in motivated behaviour to seek water and to drink it in appropriate amounts, as noted by both Adolph and Knut Schmidt-Nielsen (1964). The capacity to seek water is, however, limited and some curious things are seen. For example, desert lizards can remain well balanced solely on water content of diet and metabolic production of water. It has been found that such lizards sleeping on a rock where there was a pool of water never went to the pool, and some might die of dehydration though the water was only 3 or 4 metres away.

However, it was observed by Bradshaw of Western Australia, that when it rained the lizards, as it were, went insane. They ran around and jumped in the air, and they drank the water as it fell. In the laboratory it was necessary to have water dripping on them, and lizards would regularly come to the water and drink. The argument used by Bradshaw was that in the normal course of events the only water that desert lizards encountered was in rain. On the other hand, other lizards are pretty capable of drinking when near water, and drink regularly from it. Overall, reptiles have been shown to respond to water deprivation, i.e. cellular dehydration and also what's called extracellular dehydration due to loss of volume of the tissue fluids. They also respond to angiotensin.

Fitzsimons showed that the iguana would drink enough water after systemic injection of hyperosmotic solutions of sodium chloride to render the injected saline load equivalent to the osmotic pressure of the blood. The onset of drinking, after it was made hypertonic was quite slow. Snakes that have been dehydrated will drink in 6 minutes the amount of water of which they are deficient. It is clear that in reptiles water drinking is subserved by a much more highly organized nervous system than in fish. Most birds drink electively in response to the same stimuli that provoke drinking in mammals.

Mammals

With mammals, apart from strategies such as burrowing to avoid the heat, survival in desert in very dry conditions depends upon the thirst mechanism and resultant drinking. Humans for example under desert conditions may produce 10–15 litres of sweat in a day, with a rate exceeding more than a litre per hour. Allowing that the volume of plasma is 3 to 4 litres in a 70 kg man, the degree of stress involved in such a situation without compensatory intake is obvious. Dehydration amounting to 15–25% of body weight is fatal. After an episode of large loss of sweat, Adolph determined in his extensive studies that, when offered water, the human only corrects half or more of the deficit, and then would correct the remainder when taking food. There appears to be a limit to a very large intake in the human. On the other hand a creature such as the camel can repair very large body deficit as shown spectacularly in Schmidt-Nielsen's experiments. Knut Schmidt-Nielsen of North Carolina, is the doyen of comparative physiologists. Camels deprived of water for 2 weeks can drink up to 30% of their body weight in a single session (Schmidt-Nielsen, 1964). This can involve as much as 100 litres of water. This capacity to repair deficit with rapid drinking is characteristic of ruminant animals and has been studied in cattle, goats, and sheep. The sheep can repair body deficit following 2–3 days' deprivation of water by a drinking session lasting 3–5 minutes. The replacement is remarkably accurate.

One way or another the mammals have elaborated the mechanisms already noted. Some desert living rodents can concentrate urine to 25 times plasma concentration and thus conserve considerable water, which otherwise would be lost in excreting waste products.

Integral with these various metabolic processes involved with regulation of body fluids, Claude Bernard (1957), who enunciated the doctrine of fixité of the miliéu interiéur, recognized that it was the nervous system that was responsible for matching intake of water and of essential minerals to the loss from the body. If we consider drinking behaviour of humans it fully replaces the obligatory losses, and this goes on year in and year out. A large amount of it, particularly in Western urbanized society, is determined in the context of eating and social circumstances. The rituals include morning and afternoon tea and so on rather than being determined by physiological response to chemical changes in the body. Thus, the ritual drinking keeps the individual a little ahead before any physiological regulatory mechanisms kick in. On the other hand, Barbara Rolls and colleagues at Oxford showed that *ad libitum* drinking in dogs was determined by changes of plasma sodium concentration contingent on food intake. That is, it was determined by chemical changes in the miliéu interiéur that crossed the threshold of thirst evocation.

Medical considerations of thirst

During the last half of the nineteenth century and the first part of the twentieth century, experimental data from many sources, accompanied by logical analysis, led to the recognition that thirst was a sensation of general origin. This was stated explicitly in 1867 by Moritz-Schiff (see Fitzsimons 1979).

> Thirst being therefore above all a general sensation arising from a lack of water in the blood, and not to be identified with a feeling of dryness at the back of throat. Thirst is no more a local sensation than hunger, and the feeling of dryness in the throat that ordinarily accompanies it has only the value of the secondary phenomenon analogous to the heaviness of the eyelids which herald sleep.

The lion's share of the credit for this concept of thirst must go to the French School of Physiology, including such great figures as Magendie, Longuet, Claude Bernard, Rouleaux, Dupuytren, and Biche. The matter was clouded later by the view of the distinguished American physiologist, Walter Cannon, of Harvard. He proposed that it was the decrease of secretion of the salivary glands and the drying of the mouth that caused thirst. The lack of body water reduced the moistness of the mouth and the pharynx, and this was the seat of thirst. Aspects of this particular theory will be dealt with in the neuroimaging experiments on thirst, which I will describe in Chapter 9. Suffice to say here, the idea of peripheral origin was entertained also in the case of hunger. There was the notion that hunger arose from the contractions of the stomach, which may in fact occur. However, animals that have the stomach removed (gastrectomy) still exhibit hunger.

In relation to a number of other vegetative functions, it is clear that the feedback from the periphery can contribute to and augment the conscious state, which is, however, initiated by cerebral events. A good illustrative instance would be sexual excitation where the secondary changes that occur in genitalia and other tissues constitute sensory feedback to amplify the effect of the cerebral mechanisms that have initiated the behaviour in the first place.

In the case of thirst, other compelling knowledge pointed to the central origin. This was the fact that injection of water into the veins was able to reduce thirst dramatically even though nothing had passed through the mouth and pharynx to moisten them. There was also the evidence from clinical studies showing how tumours and lesions within the region of the third ventricle of the brain could reduce or abolish the desire to drink. Furthermore, Andersson and McCann (1955) in Stockholm, following the procedures of Hess in Zurich, showed that electrical stimulation in the hypothalamus in the region of the third ventricle could cause enormous drinking by the conscious goat. It would climb up stairs to get to the water bin when electrically stimulated.

The dry mouth theory of genesis of thirst

The attribution of thirst by Walter Cannon (1919) of Harvard to the 'dry mouth' state was historically influential. The origin of the idea was ancient and may go back as far as Hippocrates. In his Croonian Lecture in 1918, Cannon gave dubious reasons for discounting the classic experiments of Claude Bernard. Bernard had prepared a horse with a hole in its oesophagus. This is the muscular tube conveying water and food from the mouth and pharynx to the stomach. He showed that a horse with such an oesophageal fistula ejected every swallow between its front legs. Its thirst was not satisfied by massive intake of dozens of litres. It drank until fatigued and then drank again. Cannon attributed these pauses to satiation of the thirst and the recommencement of drinking to the fact that the animal's mouth dried out again. The same thing was seen with a dog with a gastric fistula, where water drunk fell out of its stomach on to the ground below. Continuous wetting of the mouth did not satisfy thirst.

Another crucial fact that should determine resolution of this issue is the consideration of a ruminant (cud chewing animal). As recounted earlier, ruminants such as sheep, cattle, and a large number of the game species of the planet have what amounts almost to a second circulation. This copious volume of fluid is produced continuously by the salivary glands. The saliva passes into the mouth and then on to the forestomach where digestion of grass occurs.

We have prepared many such animals with a permanent unilateral parotid fistula so that the secretion of one parotid gland drips continuously from the cheek to the exterior. Digestion proceeds normally with the secretion of one salivary gland going on to the forestomach. It is seen that with the withholding of access to water for 2–3 days, the severe water depletion causes a fall of rate of secretion of saliva from the one fistulated gland where the saliva is lost to the exterior. It decreases from 3 to 4 litres down to 1 litre per day. However, it indicates that the flow into the mouth from the other salivary glands, while reduced, continues and the mouth would be constantly wet. If offered water to drink the animal will drink the 3–4 litres during 3–5 minutes. This is the amount it has lost from the body in the previous 2–3 days. The thirst is satiated and interest is lost.

If, however, the animal has been prepared also with an oesophageal fistula, it will drink continuously. It may take in 10–20 litres of water over 30–60 minutes. The water drunk will pass through the already wet mouth and pharynx but then fall out of the neck before reaching the stomach. It may drink half to three-quarters its body weight of water in an hour. Thirst was not assuaged by the nearly constant passage of water through the mouth and pharynx, which was in any case superimposed on the condition of wet mouth because of continuous salivary secretion. In the human, salivary secretion is much smaller. It does, of course, decrease with dehydration. This sensation, of a dry mouth, will feed back to the brain and will add to the central chemical drive from the hypothalamic sensors reacting to change of the salt concentration of the blood. This terrible mouth dryness and sense of swelling of the tongue is a major element in the accounts of extreme thirst by survivors of shipwreck, or of being lost in the desert.

There are also other sensors in the heart and great capacity vessels, which signal reduction of volume of the circulation. These stretch receptors or 'volume' receptors send nerve impulses to the brain, which also act to augment the thirst sensation. Indeed, they may generate thirst when blood volume is lost without any concomitant change in salt concentration of blood. This occurs with bleeding such as from a stomach ulcer or a wound in battle.

Therefore, in our neuroimaging experiments where concentrated salt solution was infused into the subject's vein, a score was kept of the sensation of 'dry mouth' as well as the sensation of thirst. At the appropriate time in the sequence, the subjects were allowed to wash out their mouth with water to thoroughly wet it. However, at that stage they were not permitted to swallow. By method of difference, the activations in the brain attributable to the 'dry mouth' state disappeared after irrigating the mouth with water. This delineated the elements of the brain image attributable to the 'dry mouth'. They could be distinguished from the persisting activations attributable to the continuing central state of thirst unchanged by washing out the mouth. These disappeared immediately after drinking water and satiating thirst. As will be recounted, there were significant changes in the cingulate region after the wetting of the mouth and this ratified, to an extent, the importance of the sensory inflow from the mouth in contributing to the overall 'gestalt' of thirst sensation.

Section B—Rapid gratification of desire for water

The process of rapid satiation of thirst is a quite remarkable aspect of ingestive behaviour. There is an enormous survival advantage for a wide diversity of species in their being able to go to a water hole and rapidly correct body water deficit fairly accurately. They then quickly get out of the place. Herbivorous species are particularly vulnerable to carnivores, which may wait in the vicinity of water holes for a kill. The carnivore behaviour is emulated by hunters as recounted by Ernest Hemingway. Hunters lie in wait at a waterhole or a mineral lick.

The point at issue is that the phylogenetic development of this gratification mechanism means that, whereas gradual changes in blood chemistry are generative of thirst, the creature gratifies thirst in 3–5 minutes. Then there is a precipitate and complete decline in desire to drink. The nub of the matter is that this is long before the water drunk could be absorbed from the gut and correct the chemical deviation in the composition of the blood and fluids of the brain, which generated the thirst in the first place. The fall of sodium concentration in the blood occurs progressively over the following 15–120 minutes. The survival advantage of the neurological organization subserving this gratification behaviour is patently clear. It is an exemplar.

In the scientific records, many experiments have been aimed at teasing apart elements of the gratification process of thirst. These have included making alterations in the physiological secretory processes involved in wetting the mouth. This is contrived by using pharmacological substances to dry up salivary secretion and seeing the effect on thirst. Also, water is tubed into the stomach in water-deprived animals immediately before offering water to drink. The amount given may be equivalent to the amount of body deficit as determined by weight loss during dehydration. This can also be done before offering access to water under conditions where an oesophageal fistula is open.

The outcome emerging from the results, without describing each of these experiments in detail, is that rapid satiation is determined by a 'gestalt' of sensory inflow. The components include taste of water in the mouth, nerve impulses metering the passage of water through the pharynx and upper oesophagus ('oesophageal metering'), and nerve impulses signalling distension from filling of the stomach with water. Input from these sources is jointly sufficient and severally necessary to contrive satiation and a precipitate decline in interest. This physiological integration is clearly somehow genetically programmed. It remains very much of a mystery as to how these elements of sensory inflow *in their ordained temporal sequence* contrive within the brain the precipitate change in the consciousness of thirst with abolition of the desire for water. *It is crystal clear that the rise in salt (sodium) concentration in the blood plasma and brain fluids, which generated thirst in the first place, does not have plenipotentiary power as the concentration remains elevated for a long time after drinking has ceased.*

In terms of overall organization of integrative processes in the body, the same overall pattern is evident with other appetites—like salt appetite.

It is clearly seen with salt appetite caused by loss of sodium containing fluids from the body. Ruminant and other species of animals are genetically programmed so that on very first experience of salt deficiency they develop a specific appetite for sodium salts and can pick them out of a cafeteria of a variety of mineral salt solutions offered simultaneously in different containers.

With salt-deprived ruminant animals, when they are offered a solution of salt to drink (sodium chloride or sodium bicarbonate) they will drink in 3–7 minutes a volume of the solution adequate to provide enough salt to repair the body deficit. A precipitate decline in interest follows. This has been examined comprehensively at the Howard Florey Institute in Australia (Denton 1983). Furthermore, with sheep, if the concentration of the salt solution offered is varied, the animal adjusts volume drunk to get very close to the right amount to repair body deficiency. Thus, if the sheep has lost 600 mmol (units of salt) of sodium in 2 days, and it is offered a solution of sodium salt, which has a concentration of 900 mmol per litre, it will drink somewhere near two-thirds of a litre. If offered a solution of 200 mmol per litre it will drink nearly 3 litres. That is, in the course of the consummatory act of satiation of appetite, the animal can multiply concentration by volume and get fairly near the amount of salt to repair deficiency. That is, it integrates in its brain taste sensation signalling concentration with corresponding pharyngo-oesophageal nerve impulses metering volume swallowed. The condition under which this breaks down is when the animal is presented with a dilute solution of salt (say 100 mmol/l) and it would be required to drink, for example, 6 litres to repair deficit. Then distension of the stomach to some extent reduces the amount drunk.

Obviously the same general organization may subserve satiation of hunger. This can be seen with a dog eating its dinner, when it may be all gulps and haste, with competition between members of the pack. However, with appetite for food in humans, all sorts of cultural influences, and effects of taste (like or dislike), as well as those of concurrent drinking with resultant distension, can affect the process of gratification of appetite. Overall there is some parallel in these consummatory processes of satisfying thirst to what is seen with gratification of sexual arousal. That is, diversity of inflow via sensory channels and of psychic orientation provide a positive feedback to the central sexual appetite. This eventually culminates in orgasm, which is usually followed by an immediate and precipitate decline in desire.

Another feature of the brain organization involved in gratification of thirst is that the drinking act precipitately turns off the secretion of antidiuretic (water-retaining) hormone by the pituitary gland at the base of the brain. This, in effect, anticipates the result of absorption of water, which will reverse the effect of high salt concentration of the blood in causing antidiuretic hormone release. This has been established by Stelio Nicolaides, Jean DidierVincent, and Rougon Rapuggi, and colleagues in France, and

John Blair-West and Andrew Brook in Australia, and David Ramsay and Terry Thrasher in the USA. (See Denton 1983)

A similar thing happens with salt-deficient animals. Experiments at the Howard Florey Institute, have shown that with rapid satiation of salt appetite by drinking sodium solution, there occurs within 15 minutes a precipitate decrease in secretion of the salt-retaining hormone by the adrenal gland. This anticipates the effect of the later absorption of salt drunk. Thus, parallel with the discovery of the rapid cessation of secretion of the water-retaining hormone with gratification of thirst, these experiments (Denton 1983) on inhibition of secretion of aldosterone (the salt-retaining hormone) show the extent to which events in the mind can profoundly affect the physiological organization of the body.

Against this background let us look at what happens in the brain when a sensation of thirst rapidly invades consciousness.

Chapter 9

The neuroimaging of thirst by positron emission tomography

The experimental plan

These experiments were carried out at the Research Imaging Center in San Antonio, Texas. They involved a team from the Howard Florey Institute in Melbourne, and the Texas group led by Dr Peter Fox (see references for the personnel (Denton *et al.*, 1999b, Egan 2003)). Dr Fox has played a leading role internationally in neuroimaging.

For those readers who do not wish to follow through all the details of procedures, the salient facts were as follows.

Thirst was produced in nine healthy young male volunteers by the rapid infusion into a vein of a salt solution (sodium chloride), which was three times more concentrated than the sodium concentration of the blood.

After about 15–20 minutes of infusion, the sodium concentration of the blood plasma had increased (Fig. 9.2) and the first consciousness of thirst appeared. Neuroimaging at this point gave indication of the areas in the brain, which were activated and deactivated as a result of sensors and neurophysiological systems responding both to the change of sodium concentration in the blood, and the first emergence of consciousness of thirst.

Figure 9.1, which has several sections, will serve as a guide to the anatomical regions in the brain referred to in the text, and the location of changes that occurred in the brain during the neuroimaging experiments.

The subjects were imaged during further stages of the infusion and then again when their thirst sensation had reached maximum. This was about 40 minutes after the concentrated saline infusion was stopped. They were then allowed to rinse out their mouth with water but not swallow, and were imaged again. Following this they were allowed to drink water to satiate their thirst, and were imaged 3 minutes after they had finished drinking.

The positron emission tomography (PET) radioactive water ($H_2^{15}O$) technique detects local change of cerebral blood flow. *Activation represents increase of regional cerebral blood flow and reflects increased activity in the neurons of the local brain region. Deactivation is assumed to reflect decreased cerebral blood flow, and thus reduced neural activity in the local region.*

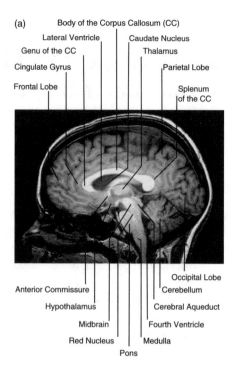

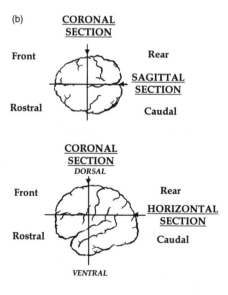

Figure 9.1 (*Continued*).

(c)

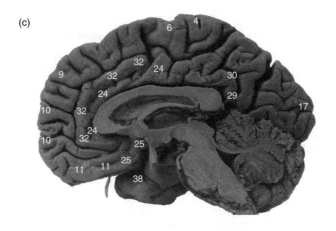

(d)

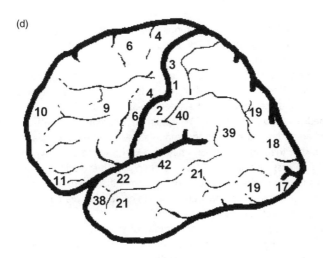

Figure 9.1 (Continued).

(e)

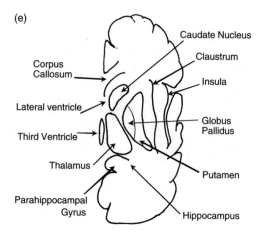

Figure 9.1 (a) A nuclear magnetic resonance (NMR) image of the brain with some of the major anatomical areas shown. The cut of this sagittal section is at the midline (see b).

(b) A diagram illustrating the use of terms in the text. Rostral = the front of the brain and caudal represents the back or rear. The lines show the direction of cut of a sagittal section (i.e. front to back), or coronal section (i.e. side to side) and the horizontal section (front to back, but at a right angle to the sagittal section). The use of the terms 'dorsal' and 'ventral' is also shown. If one considers a human body, the back is dorsal and the abdomen (the anterior)—is ventral.

(c) The medial surface of the right hemisphere of a human brain with some of the numbered areas designated by Brodmann as showing different cellular structure. It is recognized that the cortex is rather a patchwork of discrete areas. As pointed out by Northcutt and Kass, not all neural features change with evolutionary time (they are primitive characters), whereas others are highly modified (derived characters). Because of different selection pressures, the brains of living mammals are a mosaic of both primitive and derived characteristics.

(d) The lateral (outside) surface of the left lobe of the brain. Some of the areas numbered and noted by Brodmann as having particular cellular architecture are shown.

(e) A horizontal section of the brain near the level of the anterior commissure ($z = 0$) showing the claustrum, a thin long sheet of grey matter between the insula and the globus pallidus and putamen (motor structures), and the position of the parahippocampal gyrus (after Talairach and Tournoux). Because of the anatomy of the claustrum, it cannot be specifically delineated from adjacent structures (putamen and insula) by neuroimaging.

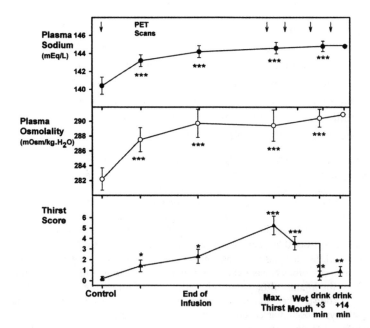

Figure 9.2 The changes in chemical composition of the blood plasma produced by rapid intravenous infusion of concentrated salt solution. The sodium concentration and osmotic pressure rose by the end of the infusion and remained increased until the end of the period of observation. The thirst score increased with the infusion and continued to increase until about 40 minutes after the infusion ended. It decreased though remaining significantly elevated, as a result of rinsing the mouth with water, which removed the 'dry mouth' component of thirst. It then fell precipitously by 3 minutes after the subjects were allowed to drink as much water as they wished (i.e. satiation).

The physical basis of this detection is that water with radioactive oxygen (^{15}O) is administered intravenously about 15 seconds before the scan. The radioactive oxygen emits positrons, which collide with electrons. This collision with annihilation of the two particles releases two photons (particles of light), which go off exactly in opposite directions. Because they are of very high energy, a significant proportion exit the skull and are detected simultaneously by a ring of radiation detectors. These are in a camera, which surrounds the head. The more cerebral blood flow in a local area increases, the more collisions. Computers create an image from these counts of collisions reflective of the changes of cerebral blood flow in local areas of the brain. The changes in neural activity are shown at the various stages of the experiment in the figures, and the proposed implications will be discussed further on.

The details of the experiment follow.

The sequence of the experimental plan

All subjects used in the experiment were normal, right-handed, non-smoking males with ages ranging from 24 to 36 years. They were asked to rate thirst, with a score of 0 for no thirst, and 10 was equivalent to the most severe thirst they could remember ever having experienced. They also rated on a scale of 0–10 any sensation that developed of their mouth feeling dry. As noted above, previous studies have shown that the sensation of thirst is generated if plasma sodium concentration or osmolality increases by about 2%.

We gave the infusion of 3% sodium chloride at the rate of about 14 ml per minute in a 70 kg individual (0.9% sodium chloride would correspond to the same sodium concentration as the blood). Two baseline scans were made before infusion began. Then after 25 minutes the first scan was made with the infusion running (see Fig. 9.2). At this point in time, plasma sodium had risen by approximately 2% and the sensation of thirst had increased from 0 to an average of about 1.5 (Fig. 9.2). That is, the subjects were just beginning to experience thirst, and, also had some sense of dry mouth.

The analysis of the data was based on method of difference. That is the neuroimages obtained when the subjects were at rest and undisturbed before infusion were subtracted from the images obtained at this early stage of infusion when thirst first appeared. Of course, when first in the scanner the brain is not inactive. Probably the subject, with eyes closed, thinks about something, and is aware of some aspect of the experimental laboratory, and this includes being aware of being in a PET scanner. However, the different ways the mind wanders would to an extent be random over the population of experimental subjects. This would be background in contrast to a consistency or uniformity of effect caused by the infusion itself as a result of both change in blood chemistry and the emergence of thirst. Thus a difference is shown by subtraction. It should be emphasized that the speed with which an image is obtained with PET (30–60 seconds) is not sufficiently rapid to pinpoint the exact instant in time when thirst first entered the stream of consciousness. The data, at best, represent the early stages of the arousal of the consciousness of thirst.

Results of imaging 25–30 minutes after start of infusion of concentrated salt solution

The scan did show very significant activations (shown in red and at a lesser intensity in yellow—Fig. 9.3 top panel). They were predominantly in the evolutionary ancient areas of the brain. These included the parahippocampal gyrus (a major cortical component of the limbic system, connecting the hippocampus (memory) and the neocortex—the parahippocampus has many types of cortical architecture including primitive cortex and is activated in many contexts of stress). Also activated were the anterior and posterior cingulate gyri (the limbic emotional system) (see Fig. 9.3), and the insula (a major visceral sensory area). There was activation also in the post-central gyrus (sensory inflow, e.g. from the dry mouth). Activation occurred in the thalamus

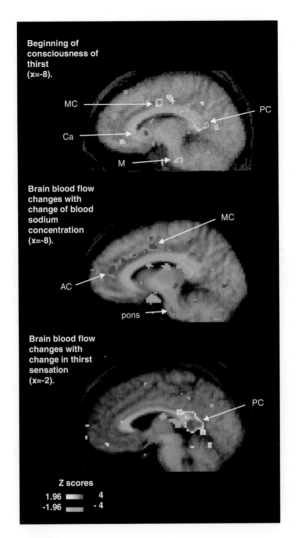

Plate 1 See page 137.

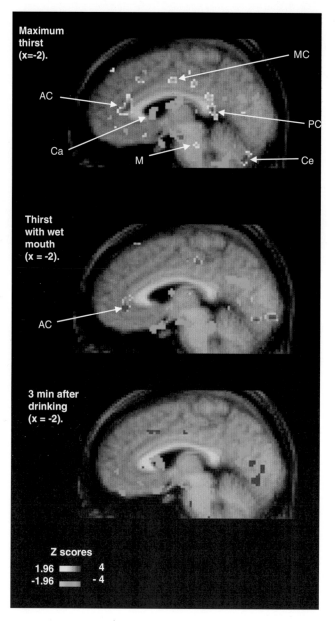

Plate 2 See page 139.

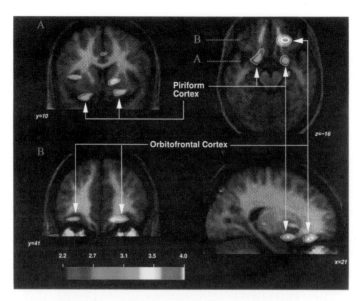

Plate 3 See page 224.

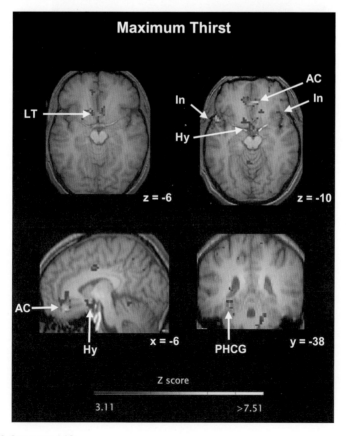

Plate 4 See page 148.

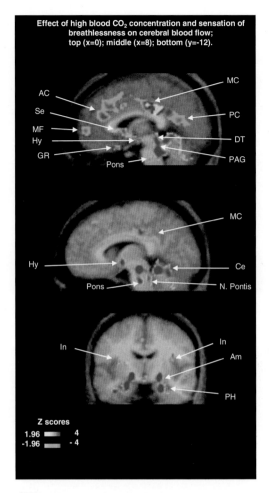

Effect of high blood CO_2 concentration and sensation of breathlessness on cerebral blood flow; top (x=0); middle (x=8); bottom (y=-12).

Z scores
1.96   4
-1.96   -4

Plate 5 See page 157.

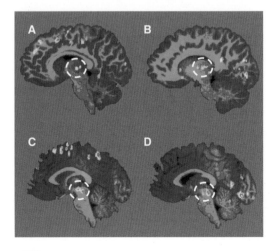

Plate 6 See page 169.

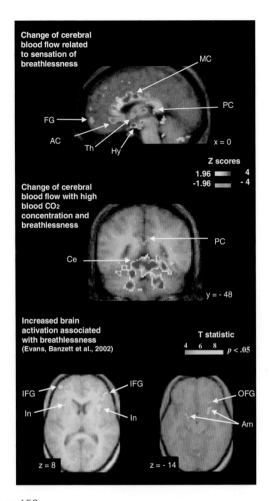

Plate 7 See page 158.

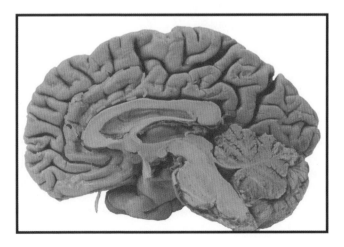

Plate 8 See page 145.

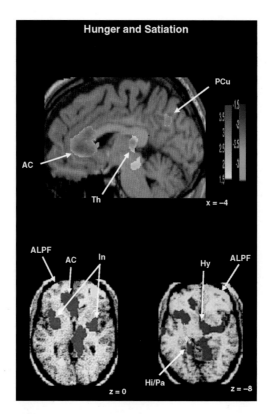

Plate 9 See page 161.

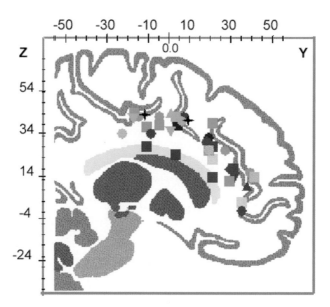

Plate 10 See page 176.

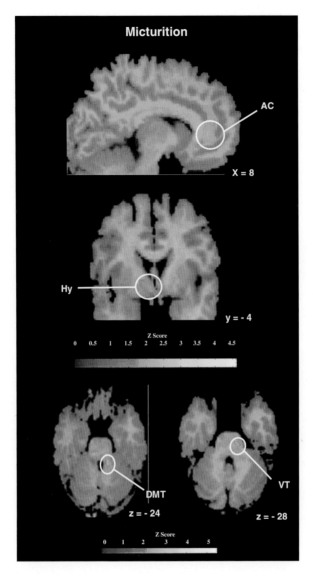

Plate 11 See page 171.

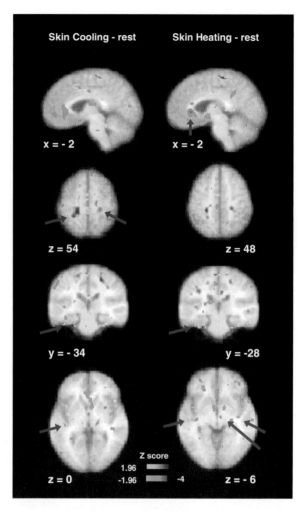

Plate 12 See page 175.

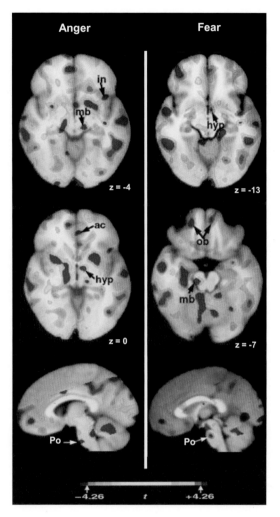

Plate 13 See page 184.

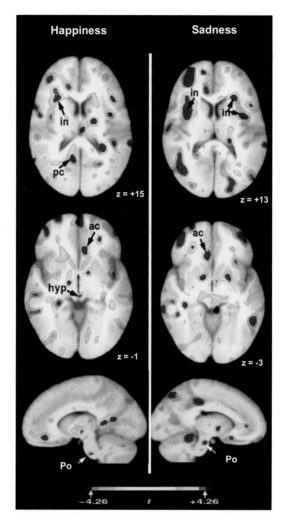

Plate 14 See page 186.

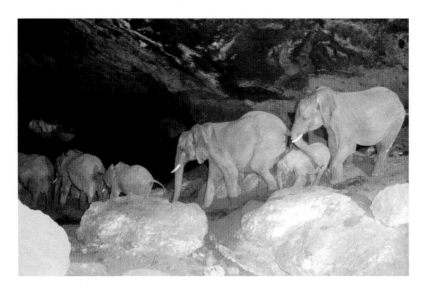

Plate 15 See page 78.

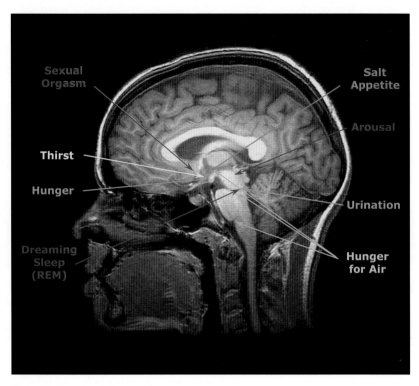

Plate 16 See page xxiv.

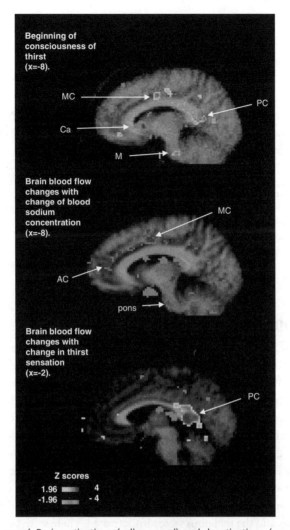

Figure 9.3 *Top panel.* Brain activations (yellow→red) and deactivations (green→blue) at a time when consciousness of thirst first appeared during infusion of concentrated saline. These are areas changed in a thin (2 mm) sagittal slice taken 8 mm from the midline on the left side. Red is more activated than yellow, and blue more deactivated than green. *Middle panel.* Areas of the brain that were activated or deactivated in relation to the rise of sodium concentration of the blood. *Bottom panel.* Brain activations and deactivations correlated with the rise and decrease of thirst sensation. PC = posterior cingulate; M = midbrain; Ca = caudate nucleus head; pons = ventral pontine nuclei; AC = anterior cingulate; MC = middle cingulate (BA 24). *Top panel:* From data in Egan *et al., Proceedings of the National Academy of Sciences USA,* **100**: 15241–15246, 2003—with permission. *Middle panel:* From Denton *et al., Proceedings of the National Academy of Sciences USA,* **96**: 2532–2537, 1999—with permission. *Bottom panel:* From Denton *et al., Proceedings of the National Academy of Sciences USA,* **96**: 5304–5309, 1999—with permission.

See also Colour Plate 1.

(relay station of sensory inflow from the periphery and pivotal in the interaction of the cortical areas and the brainstem arousal system), and in areas in the brainstem.

There was conspicuous activation also in several areas of the cerebellum. This involved substantially the evolutionary ancient parts of the cerebellum—that is down its midline. The activations in eight regions of the cerebellum actually accounted for about 13% of the total activation in the brain caused by the infusion at this point.

At this stage of the infusion, deactivations (blue for maximum, green for lesser) were seen primarily in the caudate nucleus of the brain (a motor area) and the frontal gyri and also in the cingulate, parahippocampal gyrus, and insula. There were two very strong deactivations in the midbrain and pons. The spatial accuracy of PET does not permit exact pinpointing but the deactivations may involve paranigral and parabrachial nuclei, the latter region having been implicated in genesis of salt appetite, another ingestive behaviour involving a powerful primordial emotion.

Imaging when thirst was maximal

A state of maximum thirst occurred about 40 minutes after the end of the intravenous infusion. By then the sodium concentration of plasma had risen by about 3% and the average thirst score was 5. The brain image showed areas noted at the early stage were still among the changes of blood flow, and there were, for example, stronger activations in the cingulate portion of the limbic system. Ten areas were ignited. This involved both anterior and posterior cingulate, and also six foci in the mid cingulate. Figure 9.4 (top), which represents a 2 mm wide section of the brain cut in the sagittal plane (i.e. cut from front to back) close to the midline shows a number of these cingulate activations. The most intense activation was in the parahippocampus (not shown on Fig. 9.4). The insula and the thalamus were also activated. There were 14 areas that were part of the Papez circuit (see below), which were activated above the arbitrary level of high significance. There were also activations bilaterally in the claustrum. This is a grey matter structure that lies deep in the white matter beneath the insula (Fig. 9.1e). It has extensive connections with the cingulate and the thalamus, and hypothalamus, but its function is little understood. Again, there were several activations in the cerebellum—particularly the midline vermis.

The sagittal view of the brain taken close to the midline shows clearly that the activations in the anterior and the posterior cingulate are situated close to the corpus callosum. In effect, the cingulate gyrus is like a C rotated 90° clockwise to surround the corpus callosum. The corpus callosum is the white matter traversing the middle part of the brain (see for example Fig. 9.4). It carries about 200 million fibres connecting the two sides of the brain.

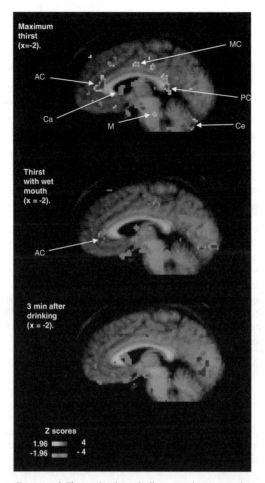

Figure 9.4 Thirst. *Top panel*. The activations (yellow→red: most activated) reflect increased neural activity and deactivations (green → blue: most deactivated) reflect decreased neural activity in discrete regions of the brain at the time when thirst was maximal (analysis of data on 9 subjects). The section is a sagittal slice (i.e. cut from front to back) and is 2 mm thick, and ($x = -2$) reflects that it is on the left side, and 2 mm from the midline. That is, it is the activity in a slice taken in the middle of the brain. The corpus callosum representing 200 million fibres joining the two sides of the brain is the large white structure that looks like a capital C rotated 90° clockwise so that its top is now near 3 o'clock. The large activation just in front of the corpus callosum is in the anterior cingulate gyrus (AC), (MC) is activation in the middle cingulate, and (PC) is activation in the posterior cingulate. Ce = cerebellum, M = midbrain, and Ca is deactivation in the region of the caudate nucleus (motor function). A large strong deactivation is seen at the top of the pons (blue). *Middle panel*. The same slice 3 minutes after washing out the mouth with water, thus eliminating the dry mouth component of thirst. The anterior cingulate activation (AC) remains, but reduction of activation in the middle cingulate in this brain slice has occurred. *Bottom panel*. The salient fact is that the large AC activation has disappeared 3 minutes after drinking water to satiation which resulted in the loss of consciousness of thirst. From Denton *et al. Proceedings of The National Academy of Sciences USA*, **96**: 5304–5309, 1999—by permission.

See also Colour Plate 2.

There were powerful deactivations in the amygdala, cingulate, and parahippocampal gyrus and thalamus. As earlier, there were very strong deactivations in the midbrain in areas that could correspond to the substantia nigra and parabrachial nucleus. The presumed reduced neural activity may be brought about by inhibitory action on the neurons caused by transmission from activated neural groups in other parts of the brain. Again, these areas affected are part of the loose construct called the Papez circuit, postulated to be involved in emotional behaviour.

Papez's (1937) notion involved the origin of emotion to be initially in the cortex with effect on the hippocampal formation (subserving memory processes) and transferral to the mammillary body in the hypothalamus. From here the anterior thalamus was excited via the mammilo-thalamic tract, and it in turn excited the anterior cingulate. Papez conceived this as the region experiencing emotion as a result of impulses coming from the hypothalamus. He also conceived that the emotive process in the cingulate could have irradiating effects on other areas of the cortex, and so add colouring to psychic processes occurring elsewhere. Papez proposed that the entire limbic lobe was implicated in the experience and expression of emotion, being the only telencephalic (rostral part of the forebrain) cortex with strong hypothalamic connections.

It is noteworthy that the highest activation with maximum thirst was in the left parahippocampus, while at the same time there were also several major deactivations in the parahippocampus. Parahippocampal neurons have been shown to project directly to the cingulate thereby bypassing the circuit proposed by Papez. Furthermore, there is a pathway continuity between the parahippocampus and the cingulate around the rear end (splenium) of the corpus callosum. Strong connections between the posterior and anterior cingulate, both of which were activated here, have been demonstrated by Vogt and colleagues of SUNY University, New York, who have pioneered much of the neuroanatomical knowledge of this limbic area of the brain. (Vogt and Gabriel 1993)
Other noteworthy areas that changed included the parietal region where the strongest activation was in the sensory regions of the mouth. This probably related to the sensory inflow from the 'dry mouth', as it disappeared when the mouth was made wet. Correspondingly, the thalamic activation could relate to transmission of sensory inflow from the dry mouth to the parietal sensory area. Flow from sensors in the hypothalamus reacting to changed sodium concentration and transmitting to cortical sites would also be involved in thalamic activation. There was also activation in motor areas (striate), e.g. in the putamen, and this could be consistent with connections from the mid-cingulate to primary motor areas with potential of mediating appropriate and immediate motor drinking responses to a disturbing situation. The insula, which was also activated, receives projections from the anterior and middle cingulate gyrus. The insula focus declined in strength with wetting of the mouth, as did the big parahippocampal activation.

Concerning the hypothalamus and midbrain, no activation in the highly relevant anterior wall of the third ventricle was seen. This may reflect the inability of the PET method to reveal any change in a very small area represented by the so-called circumventricular organs. They are small structures in the basal brain regions, which lack a blood—brain barrier, and thus respond directly to change of composition of the blood. However, as described below when the experiments were repeated using the functional nuclear magnetic resonance imaging (fMRI) method, hypothalamic activation was seen with thirst.

The purpose of recording here in some detail the anatomical regions that are functionally changed by induction of thirst was to emphasize the complexity of changes in the brain.

It could be added that some association areas of the higher cortex (particularly temporal lobe) were also changed, and these may reflect the fact that the induction of thirst very likely induced thought processes—perhaps related to the notion of satisfying thirst. Some regions of the temporal lobe are considered components of the limbic cortex. Papez (1937) described strong connections from the posterior cingulate (highly activated by thirst) to the temporal lobe of the brain. The overall pattern observed also provided a basis for comparison with the changes of loci in the brain when the next steps of the experiment were carried out. That is the wetting of the mouth to eliminate this component of the sensory inflow associated with thirst, and then the sequelae of the actual gratification of thirst by ad libitum drinking of water.

Wetting the mouth with water

Having imaged the brain at the point of maximum thirst, the subjects were then allowed to wet their mouths. This was done through a glass straw and they irrigated the mouth thoroughly with water, and spat it back out the straw without swallowing any. They had been trained previously to do this without any movement of the head or disturbance. Three minutes after this procedure the brain was imaged. Figure 9.4 (middle) shows that some areas changed as a result of the wetting. Some mid-cingulate activations disappeared though others remained. There was a reduction in the activation in the midline posterior cingulate, but another posterior cingulate area further out laterally remained (not shown in Fig. 9.4, which is a sagittal (front to back) cut near the midline). The key observation was that the area at the front of the genu—the so-called knee of the corpus callosum—in the midline persisted as a highly activated region (see Fig. 9.4—middle), as did the area in the posterior cingulate noted above. After wetting the mouth there was a lot of strong activation in the frontal lobe region of the brain. This is consistent with knowledge that has been derived from work by Professor Edmund Rolls and colleagues at Oxford (1999, 2000). They showed effects on the frontal areas of the brain during the taste process. With wetting, foci of deactivations appeared in the parahippocampus and posterior cingulate.

Drinking water to satiation

The next stage was to allow the subjects to drink as much water as they wished. Three minutes after this had been completed they were again imaged. *The striking fact was that the prominent activation area in front of the knee of the corpus callosum that had persisted with the wetting of the mouth had now disappeared—see Fig. 9.4—bottom). Thus, its disappearance was contemporaneous with the sense of gratification of thirst. That is, the consciousness of thirst was gone, as reflected by a precipitate decline of the thirst score.*

Activated areas were seen in the insula and thalamus immediately following the satiation procedure. Activations occurred also in the putamen, which is a motor area of the brain, and could have been involved in the act of drinking. At the same time there were deactivations in the posterior cingulate, insula, and the thalamus associated with this gratification. In the case of the cerebellum, there were two centres of activation with the wet mouth, and then 3 minutes after satiation six strong centres of activation were seen in older parts of the cerebellum. Following drinking, cerebellar activity accounted for 18% of the total of brain activation detected. That is, it was more active in aggregate than any other area.

Overall, the main thrust of the data was that the changes in the brain that occurred with the advent of thirst and the satiation of thirst were overwhelmingly in the evolutionary ancient areas. The findings are consonant with the concept of thirst as a primitive vegetative function with its circuitry emergent early in vertebrate evolution.

As noted above there were areas of activation in other regions—for example, the transverse temporal lobe and the cuneus (the medial surface of the occipital lobe). The implications of this are not clear, though there are connections of the cingulate, particularly the posterior, to the precuneus, hippocampus, and the temporal lobe. It may be that a pivotal primal emotion such as thirst is in humans evocative of memories of sources of fluid and the pleasures of drinking them, thus giving rise to a complex conscious experience involving association areas of the cortex. This might contribute to some activity in the temporal areas as we observed in the study.

Involvement of the cerebellum was also a striking finding. This structure had earlier on been considered to be primarily involved in the organization of movement. Lesions in the cerebellum can produce severe derangement of movement. However, in recent years brain imaging studies have indicted the cerebellum in a number of sensory processes, and also in cognitive tasks. Cerebellum involvement has been seen in the generation of words and sentences according to language rules, perceptual and spatial reasoning problems with mental rotation of objects, and with tactile discrimination. In the light of these discoveries it was of great interest to find the cerebellum was involved in a basic vegetative function such as thirst, particularly in view of the ancient evolutionary origin of the cerebellum. The comparative anatomical analysis of Butler and Hodos (1996) highlights the fact that during evolution, the emergence of jaws for capture and initial processing of prey was a major event in vertebrate history. Development of forebrain, midbrain, and hindbrain accompanied this more mobile and actively predatory life-style.

This increased mobility was subserved by development of the cerebellum in the roof of the hindbrain. Early vertebrates had only a small cerebellum or no cerebellum at all. So the evolution of jaws had a dramatic influence.

The cerebellum has many neural connections with the hypothalamus. Many of the activations with thirst were in older cerebellar regions (vermis, fastigial nucleus, and the archicerebellum to which it belongs), and these may reflect cerebellar involvement in the emotional aspects of thirst. On the other hand, as Larry Parsons (2000) of the Texas Imaging Centre has noted, those activities in the new cerebellar regions (that is the lateral hemispheres of the cerebellum) may be more related to sensory and cognitive aspects of thirst and thirst satiation. It might also be considered that the cerebellum is intrinsically involved in thirst because of the inexorable association of thirst with the intention to drink. That is, it reflects the paramount role of the cerebellum in motor activity. This intention may be closely related to expectations or plans of action, which in turn are associated with implicit or preparatory motor activity. These attributions of the nature of its functional involvement are speculative, and further experimental data are required.

As it is clearly shown in Fig. 9.3, when an analysis was made to see what areas of activation in the brain implying increased local blood flow actually correlated with the increase of sodium concentration *per se*, it was seen again that these involved primarily the cingulate regions.

A correlation was also done between the thirst score and the 99 scans done on nine subjects in this study (Fig. 9.3). In considering the comparison of correlation of images with plasma sodium concentration, and those with the thirst score, it can be noted that thirst score dropped to near zero immediately after drinking water, whereas, by contrast, the salt concentration of the blood remained elevated for some time afterwards (see Fig. 9.2) and did not fall until water drunk was absorbed in substantial quantity from the stomach. The correlation with the thirst score (Fig. 9.2) was predominantly in the posterior cingulate area (Fig. 9.3). There were also some other active areas in the anterior and middle cingulate, as seen with correlation with plasma sodium concentration. Thus, the cortical responses to both rise in salt concentration of the blood and the conscious sensation of thirst were predominantly in the cingulate regions.

Now it is well established that the cingulate is the cortical area receiving major impact from evolutionary more primitive neural regions of the brain. Twenty or more thalamic nuclei project to different parts of the cingulate cortex with the anteromedial nucleus of the thalamus having the most diffuse projections throughout this area. The cingulate area has been implicated in processes involving reward. For example, an animal will press a lever continuously for hours in order to receive small electric shocks. Self-stimulation appears rewarding for it. The cingulate is also much involved in motor function. It has more extensive projections to motor areas such as the caudate and putamen, than any other brain cortex area. Layer 5 of the cingulate has neurons that project to caudate, putamen, pons and the periaqueductal gray (PAG) of the midbrain. Output from layer 5 to motor areas may reflect hippocampal memory-based inputs that co-ordinate motor outputs related to appetite rewards.

With epilepsy of cingulate origin, intermittent psychosis or episodic outbursts are seen. Paroxysmal aggressive behaviour occurs, as well as unsociability. Often improvement has followed bilateral cingulectomy (removal of the cingulate gyrus).

With relation to the question of whether anterior cingulate lesions interfere with the thirst mechanism, there are no reports seemingly identifying a specific deficit. In cases of akinetic mutism (patients without speech or movement), there may be derangement of capacity to drink and eat, but as part of a general compromise, including incontinence. This situation follows major lesions such as rupture of anterior cerebral artery aneurysms.

An overview of the cingulate gyrus and its dominant participation in the limbic systems by Devinsky et al. (1995), recognizes an anterior (rostral) portion and a caudal part (Fig. 9.5). The rostral or front part is engaged in executive functions including those involving affect. It involves the amygdala and septum, and orbitofrontal, anterior insula and anterior cingulate cortices, the ventral striatum including the nucleus accumbens, and several brainstem nuclei including the PAG. The caudal limbic system includes the posterior cingulate cortices, the dorsal striatum, the hippocampus, and posterior parietal and posterior parahippocampus. The posterior cognitive part is involved in visuospatial and memory functions.

Parallel to these anatomical findings it has been shown by the work of Robinson and Mishkin (1968) of Bethesda, Maryland, that electrical stimulation of the anterior cingulate area in conscious monkeys caused water drinking behaviour, which to all intents and purposes simulates natural drinking. Two to eight seconds after stimulation the animals unhurriedly turned to a water spout and drank in a fashion suggesting the possibility that thirst had been evoked. This proposal was based on extensive studies of 5885 sites in the brains of 15 monkeys. It was clear that the anterior cingulate was predominantly involved. The animals sometimes took large amounts of water relative to their body mass—i.e. 400 ml over 10 minutes in a 4–5 kg monkey. The data of these authors could be consistent with the activation area of the anterior cingulate we have shown being a component in the complex pattern of activations and deactivations subserving arousal and sensation of thirst as a result of increase plasma sodium and osmotic pressure. As well as electrical stimulation, neuronal recording from this area when plasma sodium concentration is rising rapidly will be an important area of investigation for the future.

It is worth noting at this point that this effect of actual initiation of drinking by stimulating this area with electrodes contrasts somewhat with the data of Coghill and colleagues (1994) of Montreal. In the case of pain, they had the view that a distributed system subserving consciousness of it seems likely as it is very difficult to elicit painful sensations by stimulating individual local areas of the brain cortex. It may turn out that the *simultaneous* action of several regions of the brain is the necessary condition for eliciting a sensation of pain.

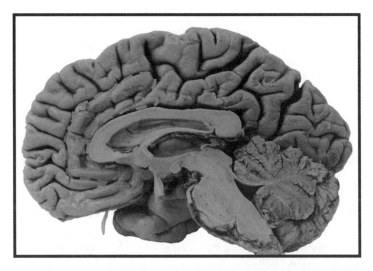

Figure 9.5 The two divisions of the cingulate gyrus as proposed by several workers. The anterior in pink is the affective area and the posterior part in green is the cognitive region.

See also Colour Plate 8.

This could also explain why discrete cortical lesions rarely lead to reduction of pain in people with intractable pain states.

In terms of integration, pathways from the mediodorsal thalamus, other thalamic nuclei and amygdala to the cingulate are well established as well as the cingulate pathway to the PAG (the arousal areas in the midbrain). It was also clear from tracer studies that neurons in the pons, which use acetylcholine as a transmitter have ascending pathways to the thalamus and these areas of the thalamus, as noted above, have widespread reciprocal connections with the cingulate area. This said, it is however, quite clear that presently very little is known about how particular structural aggregates of neurons in the cingulate area subserve particular functions. It was also important in relation to the overall considerations of brain organization that the midbrain activation we found to correlate with increase in plasma sodium was very close to the foci in the midbrain reticular formation that Per Roland and colleagues of Stockholm showed to be involved in arousal and vigilance. The midbrain reticular activity seen during the phase of rising plasma sodium concentration was the second strongest activation we recorded.

Sewards and Sewards (2000) of New Mexico, have analysed the neural organization subserving thirst. They place great emphasis on the data indicting the ventral lateral PAG as a region which in their view is the final stage of a subcortical hierarchy of structures processing the sensory signal of thirst. The outflow of signals from it go to motor areas. There is evidence of lesions in the area causing loss of thirst and stimulation causing drinking. However, similar effects occur also on food intake. They note also that stimulation in the region of the anterior wall of the third ventricle activates the ventrolateral PAG, whereas stimulation of this latter region inhibits neurons in the pre-optic area and hypothalamus. The overall view of a comprehensive analysis is that neuronal activities in the PAG contribute to awareness of thirst, and the area is a final stage in neuronal out-flow determining drinking. They cite, as strongly supporting their thesis, the data from our neuroimaging studies with intravenous hypertonic saline infusion, which show high-level activation of the PAG, particularly as related to change of sodium concentration.

Deactivations were seen in the periventricular anterior hypothalamus during change of plasma sodium concentration, and the explanation of this is not clear. As is the case of other sites of deactivations, both diencephalic and cortical, the regions do have established cingulate connections.

The cerebellum is a major part of the rhombencephalon, the hindbrain, and is an ancient part of the brain. In fact, about 70% of the neurons of the human brain are densely packed into the crystalline type microstructure of the cerebellum. The cerebellum receives input from possibly all sensory systems and projects to many areas of the cerebral cortex. The embryonic origin of it, that is the developmental origin of it (the rhombencephalon), is separate from the other brain divisions. As noted above, it has become clear over the last decade or so that it is involved in a very large number of functions over and above the participation in motor control and learned motor tasks, which traditionally have been assigned to it. Whereas some evidence has accrued for cerebellar involvement in emotional states, it becomes of prime interest to determine whether it plays a part in primal emotions of the vegetative processes. There is strong evidence of two-way connections between the nuclei and cortex of the cerebellum on the one hand, and the hypothalamus and nuclei of the thalamus on the other. The organization may be incorporated in genetically programmed behavioural patterns, the development of which came before cognitive processes involving consciousness. Thus there is a particular curiosity in the involvement of the cerebellum in response to rapidly rising plasma sodium concentration and the emergence of consciousness of thirst. In fact, it was shown also that a large part of the vermal region of the anterior central lobular region of the cerebellum was highly correlated with subjective thirst.

The cerebellum was heavily involved in response at all stages of the rise in sodium concentration, and there was also a large cerebellar activity seen 3 minutes after the satiation of thirst. There was no motor activity during the scans related to the onset of thirst, and indeed, there was no activation detected in the cortical areas devoted to motor activity except one focus 25 minutes after beginning the infusion. These data are generally consistent with the absence of motor activity or preparatory motor activity. This enforces the notion of the cerebellar findings being related in the sensation process, and it is noteworthy that a similar involvement of the cerebellum has been seen in studies of hunger.

In assigning importance to the findings in the cerebellum, it must be noted, however, that neither congenital absence of the cerebellum (its failure to develop during the development of the brain) or dysfunction as a result of damage, appear to interfere with ingestive processes, including thirst. A point emerging is that rather than the cerebellum having many different functions, in view of uniform microstructure of cerebellar tissue it is more plausible that the cerebellum subserves a fairly narrow range of functions, which can be applied generally to various kinds of neural information as permitted by its anatomical connections.

It may become highly active at times when the brain is vigilant and is monitoring its sensory receptors. Alternatively, it is plausible that the cerebellar involvement in thirst may be related to the intention to drink which is inextricably interwoven in the subjective state of thirst. The studies that have produced evidence of visceral responses in human and non-human species to cerebellar electrical stimulation and lesions, together with its reciprocal connections with the hypothalamus, support the notion that it could be involved in regulating a wide variety of visceral functions. It has also been shown that in highly aggressive monkeys, midline cerebellar lesions cause them to become more docile. It is clear that a great deal more research is needed to determine exactly how the cerebellum is involved in thirst and other vegetative behaviours as we will recount.

The fMRI imaging of thirst (functional magnetic resonance imaging)

The effects of induction of thirst by the same procedure of intravenous infusion of concentrated saline was studied with fMRI.

The basis of this technique depends on the differential magnetic properties of oxy- and desoxyhaemoglobin (i.e. whether the haemoglobin of the blood has or has not given up its oxygen). The degree to which this happens depends on the local brain activity. Therefore, alterations in the blood oxygen level dependent (BOLD) signal are used to generate maps of functional activity in the brain (fMRI).

The advantages over PET technology relate to the shorter whole brain scanning time (3 seconds) and the ability to scan continuously throughout the experiment.

The disadvantages of fMR relative to PET reside mainly in the instability of the signal if the experimental aim were to consider changes in a region over a sustained period during which a sequence of experimental manoeuvres are carried out.

Data were collected more or less continuously during the baseline period, the period of infusion, and before and after the subjects drank water to satiation. The data reported in Fig. 9.6 were collected during 10-minute periods when maximal increase of thirst sensation was experienced by the four subjects who participated in the study, and this was compared with the immediately preceding epoch to determine the areas activated by this change.

The singular feature of this study was that there was strong activation in the region of the anterior wall of the third ventricle, which includes the organ vasculosum of the lamina terminalis (Fig. 9.6). This is the site of the receptors that respond to the changes of salt concentration of the blood; i.e. surgical destruction of this area in experimental animals results in loss of thirst and absence of water drinking in response to desiccation of the body. In humans, tumours in the area can have the same effect. Overall it was important in the human imaging study to confirm activation in this region, and the technique did show up this pivotal region in the human. The activations also involved the cingulate gyrus (Fig. 9.6), and the fMR showed powerful activation in the principal regions that were shown by PET. There was strong activation of the

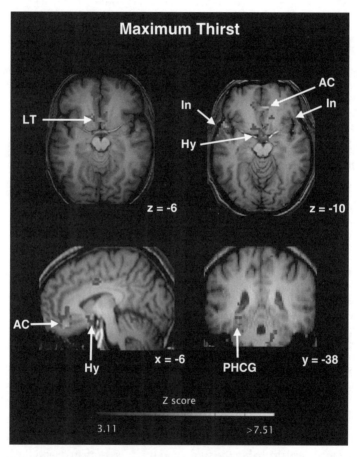

Figure 9.6 fNMR images highlighting areas of significant BOLD signal increase during the 10-minute period of maximum thirst experienced by participants. (LT = lamina terminalis, Hy = hypothalamus, AC = anterior cingulate, PHCG = parahippocampal gyrus, In = Insula).

See also Colour Plate 4.

insula in all subjects. Activation also occurred in the left parahippocampus in one subject, and in the regions of the frontal lobes.

In three of four subjects the post-central gyrus of the parietal lobe was activated bilaterally, probably related to the dry mouth sensation. Across the group several other regions were activated, including cerebellum, and cuneus, and brainstem (red nucleus region), and the mammillary bodies in the hypothalamus.

Overall the data were consistent with scientific literature on animal studies in so far as they delineated the role of the front wall of the third ventricle in the human, and they were consistent with the PET studies in terms of the cortex areas activated.

A fascinating observation emerged from this purely preliminary study. It is well worth recounting in so far as it indicates a potentially productive direction of future research.

The context is as follows. Francis Crick and Kristof Koch (1998) have stated that it seems probable 'that at any one moment some active neural processes in your head correlate with consciousness while others do not. What are the differences between them?' Discussing vision, he adds that

> it seems the brain has to impose some global unity on certain activities in its different parts, so the attributes of a single object—its shape, colour, movement, location, and so on—are in some way brought together without at the same time confusing them with the attributes of other objects in the visual field. This global process requires mechanisms that could well be described as attention, and such global unity might be expressed by the correlated firing of the neurons involved.

Edelman and Tononi (2000) discuss that at any given time only a subset of neuronal groups in the human brain—although not a small subset—contributes directly to conscious experience. The question is as to why that subset at any particular time is special, and how should the particular neuronal groups be identified? They postulate that there is a 'dynamic core', which is a cluster of neuronal groups that strongly interact among themselves, but have distinct functional borders with the rest of the brain. It is both an integrated and constantly changing composition as embodied in the term 'dynamic'. This distributed functional cluster achieves high integration through re-entrant interactions in the thalamocortical system.

With regard to Crick and Koch's (1998), and Edelman and Tononi's (2000) statements, it is cogent that the biological organization of thirst, and other specific appetites such as salt appetite, involve a capacity for very rapid satiation. The depleted animal will drink very rapidly to satiation. There is thereupon a precipitate decline in interest. Thirst disappears.

It has been noted earlier that rapid gratification of thirst has a high survival advantage.

The fMR results showed a most interesting comparison between the areas in the region of the anterior cingulate (BA32) and the anterior wall of the third ventricle. In the anterior cingulate region the signal increased during the course of the infusion, as it did also in the anterior wall of the third ventricle. The anterior cingulate signal then decreased precipitately after satiation by drinking water. This is in contrast to the activation of the lamina terminalis (part of the anterior wall of the third ventricle), which persisted with drinking (Fig. 9.7). The continued signal in the lamina terminalis area could be consistent with the fact that the raised sodium concentration of arterial blood persisted. It would only change gradually with progressive absorption of water from the gut into the bloodstream, which would be significant 10–20 minutes after drinking. Thus, the activated state in this area could be attributed directly to the changed chemical state of the miliéu interiéur caused by the hypertonic infusion, and which persisted after drinking. By contrast the activation in the anterior cingulate area could be subserving the consciousness of thirst. It would be precipitously and substantially decreased by the loss of consciousness of thirst consequent on the act of drinking water to satiation.

The observation warrants further experimental study inclusive of other areas indicted in the pattern of activation. Their precipitate decline immediately after drinking with resultant satiation may allow their delineation as a region subserving consciousness of thirst as distinct from being a region responding at a non-conscious level to chemical change in the body. That is, not all areas activated in the brain at the time of maximal thirst would be subserving consciousness of thirst. Some may be reflecting processes set in train by the increased sodium concentration in blood or be involved in neuroendocrine changes set in motion by that change in sodium concentration.

In a sense, this is addressing Crick's question. Experimental circumstance where change of conscious state is contrived by change of the chemical milieu of the body may be an apt paradigm in so far as it deals with basic vegetative systems of high survival value. The precipitate change of consciousness caused by satiation of thirst is an ideal biological context in which to identify neural aggregates subserving the consciousness of thirst.

However, the complexity of the analysis envisaged is foreshadowed by the fact that rapid satiation of thirst also turns off secretion of the water conserving hormone (vasopressin) during the act of drinking. This is a clear-cut physiological effect, involving immediate response to gratification. There are centres in the brain that regulate vasopressin secretion and presumably they would respond to gratification. This difficulty of experimental analysis may be resolved by carrying out neuroimaging experiments on humans with diabetes insipidus, a disease where there is a failure to secrete

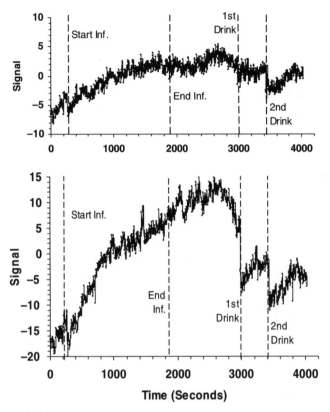

Figure 9.7 Showing the BOLD signal (fNMR) as recorded at specific locations in the brain during the sequence of the experiment. *Top*: The BOLD signal recorded in the lamina terminalis (front wall of the third ventricle region, Talairach co-ordinate 0, 0, −6) showing that the first major drink of the thirsty subject did not cause change in the signal. A small change occurred with the second drink. *Bottom*: The BOLD signal in the anterior cingulate region on the left side (−3, 33, 0) showing an increase in activation over the time course of the infusion, and then a precipitate large decline in the signal following drinking water to satiation. The second drink also caused decline.

vasopressin—the water conserving hormone. The neuroimage with gratification can be compared with gratification in normal humans, which might identify those areas involved in vasopressin secretion. It is an interesting future experimental area.

Chapter 10

Neuroimaging of other primordial emotions, and also the second level distance receptor evoked emotions

Some of what was found with the neuroimaging of thirst was predictable from earlier knowledge of neurophysiological and neuroanatomical systems involved in thirst. Some things were novel. It is evidently cogent to the hypothesis being advanced to consider the neuroimaging data of other primal emotions.

With relation to what is to follow, the lay reader will soon be aware of the complexity—the multiplicity of regions involved—with different emotions. *The essential fact emerging from the chapter is that the primordial emotions cause major changes in the evolutionary ancient areas of the brain as did our exemplar—thirst.* Rather than become immersed in a description of the various anatomical regions, which may have particular implications for those with a knowledge of neuroscience, the lay reader may note some general issues of scientific interest in the overall context, but might find it easier to pass over the sections with boxed text. Continuity of the theme of the book will not be lost.

Breathing

Hunger for air—breathlessness—is the outstanding example of an imperious sensation with compelling intention—which is to breathe. It can give rise to a sense, as the Harvard respiratory physiologist Banzett points out 'of feeling you are going to die.'

Ordinarily, breathing or respiration goes on in all of us beyond the realm of consciousness. Only occasionally do we become aware of it. It can reflect the gradation of sensation. First, an awareness of the process of hitherto unconscious breathing, then a wave of strong desire and need to breathe, climaxing with a tsunami—a completely overwhelming sensation. Breathlessness or 'air hunger' is a dominant and very distressing symptom of a number of common and dangerous illnesses. These include heart failure, and emphysema, which usually develops as a result of smoking. It occurs in other lung diseases such as asthma.

The control of respiration is by nerve cell groups in the medulla, a part of the ancient hindbrain. There are attested pathways from this primary respiratory control group that go to other brainstem, midbrain, cerebellar, hypothalamic, thalamic, amygdala and hippocampal and insular regions. This has been shown by pathway tracing techniques. Thus, it was likely such regions might show up with neuroimaging experiments where a state of breathlessness was created—They did.

These hindbrain neural groups provide the primary oscillatory control of breathing in mammals (that is, the neurones oscillate automatically). However, they react to change in the carbon dioxide (CO_2) concentration of the arterial blood which supplies them. This determines the acidity of the fluid milieu around the cells of this control system. The cells are exquisitely sensitive to change of acidity. The milieu becomes more acidic with higher CO_2 content of blood. The oscillator also responds to nervous input when, for example, the lungs are damaged or not functioning normally. Lower down in the evolutionary tree as with fish and amphibians, respiration is controlled in response to reduction of the oxygen content of blood. However, with mammals a rapid response system reacting to blood CO_2 has evolved.

In relation to control of respiration by higher centres of the brain, brain imaging has shown that voluntary control of breathing—that is, for example, increasing the pace of breathing by an act of will—is associated with activation in the motor cortex. This might be expected. However, independently of such volition, intense breathlessness can occur in certain psychiatric states such as panic disorder. It is theorized that this is due to malfunction of the suffocation alarm. There appears to be no physiological malfunction to account for this reaction.

Guz (1997), a UK leader in the study of control of respiration, working with the distinguished Queens Square group in London, led by Frackowiack and Friston, and also with Colebatch, Adams and Corfield at the Charing Cross and Westminster Medical School, has pointed out that it is not the output of nerves to the muscles of breathing that give rise to the hunger for air. The key is the intact brainstem oscillator. Consistent with this, Simon Gandevia and colleagues (1993) of Sydney, and Banzett and colleagues (1990), have shown mechanically ventilated subjects who have been paralysed by curare (a South American arrow poison that blocks activation of muscles by motor nerves) report severe air hunger when the CO_2 concentration in blood is increased. This is done by increasing the concentration of

CO_2 in inspired air. Similarly, in quadriplegics (lesions in the upper cervical spinal cord) increased arterial CO_2 causes severe air hunger, though the motor pathway from the brainstem to motor cells of the respiratory musculature in the spinal cord is interrupted. Data on the terrible 'locked in' brain syndrome highlight that there are presently unknown elements in respiratory control. In this syndrome all sensory input to the brain is intact, but a lesion in the pons and lower midbrain destroys motor transmission. Thus the patient's voluntarily control of muscle movement is abolished with the exception of the capacity to raise the eyelids. Though breathing is normal and regular, a voluntary effort to change the rate has no effect. However, it can be shown that the patients become breathless with increased CO_2 in inspired air. Also, of great interest, emotion will disrupt breathing. This suggests that perhaps unknown pathways exist from areas of the cortex (presumably limbic areas associated with the emotion), which would be anatomically separate from the main pathway from the cortex to the brainstem. This main pathway from the cortex can influence the respiratory oscillator in the brain medulla, but it will have been divided by the lesion.

Guz (1997) says we really are at an early stage only of our understanding of how higher brain centres control respiration. He suggests we don't really know how a human can take a breath at will, or how expiratory airflow can be perfectly controlled to produce speaking or singing. Nor, he says, can we explain how breathing increases the right amount during exercise. There would not seem to be an error signal to regulate breathing in the absence of the metabolic acidosis that occurs with severe exercise.

Neuroimaging of breathing

For the purpose of experiments on neuroimaging, a rise of rate of respiration together with severe hunger for air can be produced easily by increasing the CO_2 of the air breathed from the usual atmospheric concentration of 0.1% up to 8%. Brain imaging experiments using increased CO_2 to produce breathlessness were carried out in 1991 by the London group referred to above. They identified activations in brainstem, hypothalamus, thalamus, and extending up to the limbic system as evidenced by activation in parahippocampus, hippocampus, anterior cingulate, and insula, and the fusiform gyrus. The latter is a part of the temporal lobe of the brain. The results indicated, therefore, participation of the limbic system in the complex situation of *the concurrent effect of high blood CO_2 together with the subjective sense of air hunger*. The authors suggested the activations and deactivations were set in motion by both causes. The onset of breathlessness with increased CO_2 is rapid. Sensors in the medulla detect the rise of arterial blood CO_2 (termed hypercapnia). As effects of the two processes, high blood CO_2 and breathlessness, are not easily distinguishable, an important experimental aim was to identify the particular neural activations and deactivations that are involved specifically in consciousness of breathlessness.

Accordingly, as part of the experiments made in the year 2000 at the Research Imaging Center in San Antonio, Texas, by a team of US and Australian scientists, CO_2 was administered to healthy young human volunteers in one of two ways. One method was by a face mask. An alternative method was by a mouthpiece. The volunteers found breathing through a mouthpiece was much easier than breathing through a face mask. It was contrived that the CO_2 administered in the two modes resulted in similar blood CO_2 content. This was validated by CO_2 analysis of expired air. However, there was considerably less sense of breathlessness with the mouthpiece administration. Subtraction of the mouthpiece scan from the face mask scan revealed the neural changes specific to the consciousness of breathlessness as the CO_2 content of blood was the same in the two instances.

Concurrent action of high blood carbon dioxide and breathlessness

First however, let us consider the data on the effect on the brain when the two processes—hypercapnia (high blood CO_2) and breathlessness acted together. Figure 10.1 shows that the effect was dramatic. The field of scan did not take in the medulla so that the respiratory oscillator neural centres did not show. However, as might have been expected from the known pathways traced from the medulla, very powerful activation occurred in the midbrain tegmentum (in the dorsal or back part of the midbrain) (Fig. 10.1). Also, the periaqueductal gray was activated (the region in the centre of the midbrain surrounding the canal extending between the third ventricle in the hypothalamus and the fourth ventricle in the medulla (Fig. 9.1a)). A pons area was also activated as well as a centre in the posterior hypothalamus. Many limbic areas were ignited including the amygdala, the hippocampus, the parahippocampus region at several sites, and the anterior cingulate, the insula and the fusiform gyri of the temporal lobe. There were also motor areas as represented by the caudate nucleus and putamen of the striate complex (Fig. 10.1 shows some of these in the 2 mm (millimetre) slices of the brain that are represented in the figure.)

Very striking deactivations also occurred. These deactivations occurred in dorsal anterior cingulate, and the posterior cingulate (Fig. 10.1). There were also relatively massive deactivations seen in several sites in the middle frontal gyrus as well as in the orbital gyrus and the gyrus rectus. These latter two gyri are on the undersurface of the frontal lobe. There were massive activations in the cerebellum (16 areas ignited—Fig. 10.1) and nearly all were within 25 millimetres of the midline and thus in the evolutionary more ancient part of the cerebellum.

Air hunger or breathlessness

When the subtraction analyses noted above (i.e. facemask minus mouthpiece) were made to define *the activations attributable to the consciousness of air hunger alone*, the pattern of activations and deactivations were different. The singular feature was that air hunger caused activations predominantly in the limbic system of the brain—particularly the anterior cingulate gyrus on both sides (Fig. 10.2), the insula and claustrum, the amygdala, and also the thalamus, hypothalamus, and periaqueductal gray. Areas in the temporal lobe and

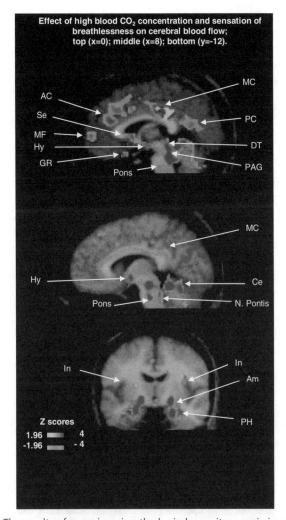

Figure 10.1 The results of neuroimaging the brain by positron emission tomography (PET) during a physiological state when both blood CO_2 concentration was raised and a strong hunger for air (breathlessness) was experienced in nine subjects. *Top panel* (A sagittal section in midline, x = o) shows powerful activation (red–yellow) in the midbrain tegmentum (MT) and the periaqueductal gray (PAG), the cerebellum (CE) and the hypothalamus (Hy). There was powerful deactivation of areas (green–blue) in the anterior cingulate (AC) and the posterior cingulate (PC) and the medial frontal cortex (M) and gyrus rectus (GR). The sagittal section—*middle panel* (x = 8), which is further out on the right shows the dorsal tegmentum (DT), pons, and posterior hypothalamus (Hy) activations. The coronal section—*bottom panel* (y = −12) shows strong activations in the amygdala (AM) and parahippocampal regions (PH), and activations in the insula (IN). From Brannan *et al.*, *Proceedings of the National Academy of Sciences USA*, **98**: 2029–2034, 2001—with permission. See also Colour Plate 5.

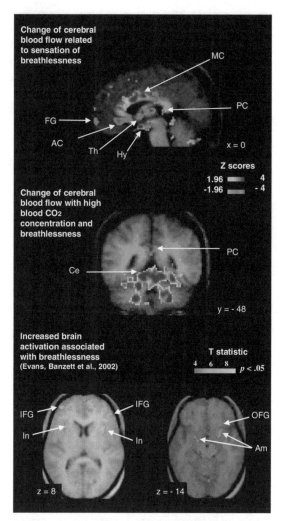

Figure 10.2. *Top panel.* The effect of breathlessness (air hunger) alone showing activation in the middle cingulate (MC), posterior cingulate (PC), hypothalamus (Hy), and cerebellum. There was large deactivation in the anterior cingulate (AC), frontal lobes (FG) and the thalamus (Th). (From Liotti *et al.*, *Proceedings of the National Academy of Sciences USA*, **98**: 2035–2040, 2001.) *Middle panel.* A coronal section of the brain showing the massive activation in the cerebellum (Ce) with the combined effect of high arterial blood CO_2 and breathlessness. (From Parsons *et al.*, *Proceedings of the National Academy of Sciences USA*, **98**: 2041–2046, 2001.) *Bottom panel.* A study of breathlessness by Banzett's group at Harvard, showing a major role of the insula (In), and also activations in the inferior frontal gyrus (IFG), orbitofrontal gyrus (OFG) and the amygdala (Am). (From Banzett *et al.*, *Journal of Neurophysiology*, **88**: 1500–1511, 2002—with permission.)

See also Colour Plate 7.

lingual lobe were activated also. Strong deactivations were seen in the frontal gyri, thalamus, and the striate (motor) nuclei.

When a different type of analysis was done to directly determine what changes in the brain actually correlated (i.e. matched or moved with) with the subjective sensation of breathlessness, the effects were predominantly in the cingulate, insula and claustrum, and also the temporal and lingual gyri. Overall, the effects were in the evolutionary ancient areas of the brain, as with thirst.

An outstanding well controlled experiment to distinguish the effect of air hunger from that of raised blood CO_2 was made by Banzett *et al.* (Harvard School of Public Health) in 2000. Subjects were positive pressure ventilated with a nose mask or mouthpiece. The volume and rate of ventilation could be directly controlled. If the volume of respiration was experimentally restricted to be below what would have occurred spontaneously with a particular level of CO_2, then severe air hunger was produced. Imaging showed the major activations were in the right insula with lesser ones in the left insula. That is, with CO_2 concentration constant, the insula was indicted as a predominant locus of the emotion of hunger for air. The insula appears to be a very important integrating structure for behaviours associated with homeostasis.

Recently, Evans and Banzett (2002) of Harvard, together with the London Group of Adams, Frackowiak, McKay and Corfield, have made the first functional nuclear magnetic resonance (fNMR) study of air hunger. This gave better spatial resolution. The subjects were mechanically ventilated and air hunger was produced by reducing the tidal volume of respiration. This obviated the global increase of cerebral blood flow contingent on increasing blood CO_2.

The salient feature of the results was the activation of the anterior insula (Fig. 10.2). It extended from the granular superior field, through the transitional dysgranular field to the inferior agranular field of the insula. On the right side the insula activations were confluent with activations in the frontal regions. This involved superior, inferior, and middle frontal gyri. There were also major activations in the anterior cingulate, and in the phylogenetically ancient regions of the cerebellum. Activations occurred in the intraparietal sulcus, the amygdala, and putamen.

The authors draw attention to the commonality of the finding of the activation of the insula in this and previous primal emotion studies—e.g. thirst. They emphasize its wide connections, as attested by neural pathway tracing, particularly to the motor centres controlling breathing. The insula has both afferent and efferent connections with all neighbouring limbic centres activated in the study—anterior cingulate, operculum, thalamus, orbital frontal cortex, amygdala, and basal ganglia. Other studies have shown that the insula is involved in distressing stimuli with negative emotional valence (hunger). Also, the activation of the amygdala in this and earlier studies is consistent with the aversive nature of breathlessness.

The overview of the authors appears to be that the insula has something of a plenipotentiary role in a network giving rise to the consciousness of breathlessness. In their discussion, they note, also the predominance of phylogenetically ancient areas of the brain in the network subserving breathlessness, an emphasis consonant with the theme of this book.

James Augustine (1996) of the University of South Carolina has emphasized the complex role of the insula as a sensory area with many facets, and as a visceral motor area. Peyron and colleagues (2000) of St Etienne and Lyon in France, have described data showing the intensity of pain involves the anterior insula, the secondary sensory cortex and the thalamus on the opposite side. However, the *attention* to pain involves the anterior cingulate, both thalami and the posterior parietal and prefrontal cortices.

Considering the cerebellum again, it was the ancient midline area that was activated by air hunger—the central lobule and the culmen. Activity in the central lobule showed it was also the main region to correlate with the intensity of air hunger.

The pattern of data fits with experimental studies that show cerebellar involvement in other functions driven by internal sensors, both vegetative and autonomic. That is, functions such as input from blood vessels, visceral pain, thirst as described above, and hunger for food. Furthermore, in the case of the compelling primal emotions, hunger for air, thirst, pain, and hunger for food, the pattern of cerebellar lobules activated was similar.

Whereas the cerebellum has been deeply implicated in motor functions since the first studies of it were made, there was no evidence in our imaging scans that activation in the motor areas of the cortex of the brain occurred with hunger for air and hypercapnia. However, as intention to breathe, to gain access to air, is an inherent element in the conscious state evoked, it may be that the intention or expectation involves implicit or preparatory motor activity that could activate systems in the cerebellum supporting motor behaviour.

Commonality of brain elements subserving the primordial emotions

Let us now consider some primordial emotions other than thirst and hunger for air. These include hunger for food, pain, desire to pass urine, and the compelling desire to sleep, and changing body temperature—both skin and core, and sexual orgasm. There is some measure of congruence between the loci of activations and deactivations that are seen vis à vis those with thirst. That is, the general anatomical areas involved were similar, though whether they were activated or deactivated sometimes was different.

Food hunger

Food hunger was studied by Tataranni and colleagues (1999) of Phoenix, Arizona. Hunger elicited by 36 hours of fasting caused a pattern of activation with similarities to thirst. There were activations in the anterior cingulate (Fig. 10.3), the insula, claustrum, the hippocampus, and parahippocampus (all ancient areas of the forebrain), and in the hypothalamus, and in the motor

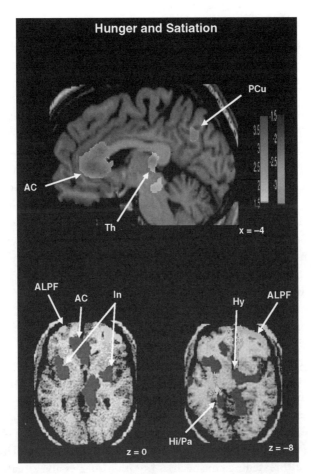

Figure 10.3 *Top panel.* A sagittal positron emission tomography (PET) image of the brain involving comparison of 36 hours hunger with satiation. A large activation is seen in the anterior cingulate area (AC), and in the thalamus (Th) and the precuneus (PCu). (Figure kindly prepared by Tataranni *et al.*, from data published in *Proceedings of the National Academy of Sciences USA*, **96**: 4569–4574, 1999.) *Bottom panel.* Brain regions with significant activation with hunger are shown in blue (AC = anterior cingulate, In = insula, Hy = hypothalamus, Hi/Pa = hippocampus/parahippocampus). Brain regions activated with satiation are shown in yellow (ALPF = ventrolateral prefrontal cortex). (From Tataranni *et al.*, *Proceedings of the National Academy of Sciences USA*, **96**: 4569–4547, 1999.)

See also Colour Plate 9.

nuclei represented by the caudate and putamen, as well as in the cerebellum. There was also activation in the posterior orbitofrontal and anterior temporal cortex, and the precuneus (the precuneus has connection to the posterior cingulate gyrus).

Pain

Pain is a powerful primary emotion, which if severe may expel any other perceptions from the stream of consciousness. It may arise from structural damage to the external surface of the body or, it may come from structures deep within the body. Examples of the latter would be the pain from anoxia of the heart muscle with angina or coronary occlusion, or from an internal ulcer or inflammation irritating the peritoneum of the abdomen. A blow to the testicles is a particular example of internal pain.

Grover Pitts (1994), Emeritus Professor of Physiology, University of Virginia, USA, has contributed an outstanding essay on the evolutionary aspects of pain, and I will follow closely his line of thought here. He suggests pain is understood by both layperson and clinician as conscious suffering. A behavioural definition is that it is a phenomenon characterized by withdrawal or flight in any animal, vertebrate or invertebrate. It is recognized that it is acute pain that usually evokes such behaviour. However, with 'slow' pain, inactivity may be the demeanour that is conducive to recovery.

Pitts (1994) cites Homer Smith's statement that consciousness, (1) keeps the brain's 'sensory screen aglow' during intervals between consecutive sensory stimuli. This gives rise to a time dimension, (2) it allows integration of present with past (memory), and prediction of future, (3) it permits individual choice between alternatives of action. Pain is perceived only during consciousness. Consciousness allows processing of pain stimuli along these lines. *Absence of consciousness would render memory and the integration process virtually useless, and largely delete the survival value of pain.* Pitts sees these as facts of massive evolutionary significance. This is because creatures can memorize a large portfolio of threatening conspecifics or, other species and situations, and avoid them before damage and pain becomes inevitable.

William James (1890) gave a succinct overview on the utility of consciousness. He stated that the empirical connection between subjective feelings of pain and objective injury on the one hand, and between feelings of pleasure and life enhancing activities could only be explained if evolution had rendered subjective states effective in adapting animals to their environments. That is, if consciousness had not served some useful purpose it would not have evolved. With humans, of course, speech allows cogent information on these issues to be transmitted from generation to generation.

In deducing the existence of pain in species other than our own, the behavioural criterion of avoidance and withdrawal is paramount. With many species they do vocalize—cry out. A sound emitted by an animal like a scream might well indicate experience of pain in particular circumstances. However, chimpanzees, for example, scream for more than one reason. Grover Pitts

(1994) suggests criteria for the existence of pain in animals might be seen in three categories. First is the structure of the nervous system, second is comparative brain size, and the third is behaviour. The capacity to experience pain appears dependent upon a specific neural organization in the brain and spinal cord in a fashion similar to other sensory systems such as touch or hearing.

Thus, Pitts (1994) sees it as a cogent point, that the spinoreticular–thalamic system, which carries pain fibres from the periphery to midbrain and thalamus, is conspicuous in vertebrates at the level of fish, amphibians, and reptiles, just as in a wide variety of mammals studied. Of the central structures of the pathway, the reticular system is present in all vertebrates, as are some components of the limbic system. There are pain pathways in addition to the spinoreticular systems. Overall a reasonable summary statement according to Pitts is that neural structures believed to be associated with pain are widely represented in mammals and in some birds, reptiles, amphibians, and fish.

Pitts proposes that as consciousness is necessary for experience of pain, a brain size adequate to experience consciousness and memory is necessary for pain. Thus a decrease of central nervous system (CNS) size may reach a point where it is too small. The size should not be too sharply defined. Marian Stamp Dawkins (2000), of the Zoology Department at Oxford University, remarks 'That judgement of capacity to experience pain in animals should not emphasize their cognitive abilities since it does not take much intellectual effort to experience pain, fear, or hunger'. However, the mass of the CNS over the range of vertebrates from humans down to goldfish varies from 1000- to 10 000-fold. At the lowest level, pain may be attenuated, intermittent, or absent.

It is interesting to contemplate this lowest level in terms of the stimulus to trout behaviour when they are hooked through the mouth by a fisherman using a fly or a metal lure. As any fly fisherman knows they swim rapidly, jump and, in particular, shake their heads vigorously and sometimes dislodge the fly hook. It is conjectural whether the line and hook obstructs their intention to swim in a particular direction to a safe place, and their repertoire of reaction is an exaggerated form of a pre-programmed reflex behaviour. This might, perhaps, be related to the normal circumstances of their moving upstream against obstacles such as rocks and swift current with jumping behaviour or swimming to a place under a rock. But it is, at least, possible that it is a behavioural response to pain, as distinct from genetically transmitted reflex behaviour that happens to be coincidentally conducive to escaping lures—or it is both.

With invertebrates, the view of Pitts (1994) is that they do not have the neural organization seen in vertebrates, and the brains are too small. Further, they have sequentially arranged ganglia as distinct from true centres. Such widely spaced components are most unlikely to support functions such as memory, integration processes, and pain, which are centralized and, certainly, in the case of pain, involve consciousness. As in the main they have short lives, there would be little opportunity to apply the benefits of past experience of pain, and this would greatly decrease any survival value of pain perception in invertebrates.

The great exception to this group of suggestions may be the octopus, which has a large brain with correlation centres as was discussed earlier in Chapter 4. J.Z. Young (1964) points out that pain fibres go to the verticalis lobe, which has 150 million neurones. Learning based on electric shock to a tentacle is evident in the octopus, and it does not have to learn it eight times. Pitts (1994), while emphasizing the uncertainty of data in the animals with small brain size, and the invertebrates, notes that the octopus has evolved an eye comparable with the vertebrates. It may have independently evolved the capacity for conscious processes, memory, and pain.

With neuroimaging of pain, the studies with PET and fNMR have shown involvement of the secondary somatosensory cortex, the cingulate gyrus, and the frontal cortex. Also subcortical structures such as those in the midline midbrain, thalamus and in the motor system (lentiform nucleus) and the cerebellum are involved.

With relation to these findings, the evidence indicates that the postcentral gyrus immediately behind the big central fissure or sulcus of the brain (Fig. 10.4), which is called S_1 (somatosensory cortex), gets the first input via the thalamus. The thalamus has transmitted the pain signals from the peripheral nerves. The part of the gyrus which lights up is determined by the part of the body (e.g. the leg) where the painful stimulus was applied. Thus activity is largely on the side of the brain opposite to the origin of the painful stimulus. That is the pathway bringing the stimulus from the periphery like the leg, crosses to the opposite side low in the brain so the activation is in the hemisphere opposite to the site of stimulation. However, effects in the secondary somatosensory cortex (S_2) predominate. These activations occur on both sides of the brain. The secondary somatosensory area is around the Sylvian or lateral fissure at the bottom part of the S_1 somatosensory cortex (Fig. 10.4). It lies along the upper bank of this big lateral sulcus and includes the operculum. These pain processing areas are very superficial, and the magnetic fields associated with their activity can be easily detected using the superconducting quantum interference device (SQUID), which operates at temperatures of, for example, $-269°C$.

The PET studies of pain by the group at the Montreal Neurological Institute, including Coghill *et al.* (1994), showed pain, due to heat applied locally as, for example, to a leg, activated both sensory areas S_1 and S_2. The anterior cingulate and anterior insula, the supplementary motor area and putamen, basal part of the thalamus and claustrum were activated also. There was deactivation

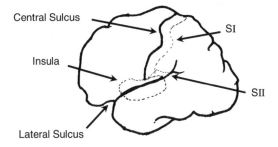

Figure 10.4 A diagram of the lateral surface of the left hemisphere showing the two great fissures of the grey matter surface (the lateral sulcus and the central sulcus). The primary somatosensory area (SI) lies along the caudal side of the central sulcus and the secondary somatosensory area (SII) runs along the upper surface of the lateral sulcus near where it joins the central sulcus, and the walls of the lateral sulcus above are the operculum—literally the lid.

of the posterior cingulate. Thus again, the limbic areas were mainly involved. All pain studies show activity of the anterior cingulate, which receives its information from the spinothalamic tract, which conducts most of pain input.

An important finding of the Montreal group was that if perceived intensity of pain was reduced or increased by hypnosis, it was shown that increased perceived intensity was associated with increased activity of the anterior cingulate areas.

In an analysis of pain, which is similar in regard to both biological overview and terminology to that taken in this book, A.D. Craig (2000) of Phoenix, Arizona states that converging evidence compels a new specific view of pain as a homeostatic emotion akin to temperature, itch, hunger, and thirst, and also visceral distension, and muscular ache. He says that 'emotions consist of a sensation and a motivation, and (therefore) pain is one of the distinct homeostatic emotions that directly reflect the condition of the body.' Just as all animals thermoregulate, all vertebrates respond similarly to the noxious stimuli that can cause feelings of pain in humans. The neural basis of these integrated homeostatic emotional behaviours must be evolutionarily ancient. *Pain in humans is a homeostatic emotion reflecting an adverse condition in the body that demands a behavioural response.* He sees it as involving a distinct sensation in the interoceptor driven regions, including the anterior insular cortex, which he terms the feeling self. Also, it results in affective motivation engendered in the anterior cingulate cortex, which is the agent of behaviour.

The thalamus and the waking state

Mircea Steriade (1987) of Laval University, Quebec, Canada, a leading authority on the thalamus, notes that the neurones of the thalamus operate in two opposite ways. This will have profound effects on the cortex. This is because they reflect two distinct behavioural modes. The *relay* mode is the characteristic of the waking state. The neurones exhibit tonic sustained firing, and high fidelity transmission of incoming messages going up to the cortex. There is efficient responsiveness with reliable synaptic transmission. Steriade puts it that there is input selection through inhibitory sculpturing and output timing. On the other hand, the *oscillatory* mode marks the resting behavioural states, particularly drowsiness and slow wave sleep. Burst electrical discharges are interspersed then with long periods of neuronal silence associated with depressed transfer function. Thus, what goes on in the cortex depends to a large extent on these alternating modes of thalamic function.

Slow wave sleep, as indicated by the name, is associated with an electroencephalograph (EEG) record of large stereotyped waves at about 1–4 per second. It is dreamless sleep. Awakening from a slow wave sleep coincides with depolarizing influences on neurones, which, therefore, block the slow wave oscillations. The EEG changes from its synchronization to desynchronization. This allows full responsiveness to output from elements of the thalamus. The arousing influences on the thalamocortical systems start from the midbrain reticular formation. The neurones in this brainstem area project to the thalamus where they excite the thalamocortical cells. The discharge rates of the midbrain reticular cells increase significantly about 10–15 seconds prior to the earliest signs of EEG desynchronization and behavioural arousal—i.e. waking up.

It remains something of a conundrum that sleep with rapid eye movements (REM) (this is EEG desynchronization sleep when dreaming occurs) is quite similar to wakefulness. Steriade says the two are similarly brain activated states embodying a response readiness. They receive external stimuli when awake, or internal drives when dreaming. Conversely, when going to sleep the RAS slows down its discharge rate to the thalamus. Transmission through the thalamic cortical neurones diminishes dramatically with onset of EEG synchronization—well before behavioural indications of sleep. This deprives the cortex of input required to elaborate a response. In effect, it deafferents (closes off input to) the cortex as a prelude to falling asleep.

All told, there are over 30 nuclei (particular populations of neural cells) in the thalamus. The three major types can be recognized:

1. The relay nuclei receive incoming signals involved in sensory and motor processing. They project to the cortical layers IV and III. The lateral geniculate, which relays impulses from the retina of the eye, is highly organized, and the ventral posterior nucleus receives sensory signals on the way to the somatosensory cortex. Other nuclei deal with auditory input or motor signals.

2. The intralaminar nuclei, which lie between the medial and lateral nuclei, receive input from diverse sources in the body—motor centres, pain pathways, and arousal systems (Fig. 11.2). They project to the forebrain and to layer I and layer VI of the cortex in widespread fashion.

3. The reticularis nucleus is a thin sheet surrounding the thalamus and does not project to the cerebral cortex (Fig. 11.2). However, all thalamocortical and corticothalamic axons pass through it and contact its neurones. It thus influences thalamic activity and is a key structure in this regard. Francis Crick (1984) has synthesized evidence from behavioural and electrophysiological experiments to support the existing

hypothesis that the brain's internal attentional searchlight is controlled by the reticular nuclei of the thalamus, which is rather the gateway to the cortex. This is done by production of rapid bursts of firing in the region of the reticular complex, which corresponds to the most active part in the thalamocortical maps, and this process is subserved by cells with particular properties of their synapses.

A number of theories of consciousness involve corticothalamic and thalamocortical loops, also embodying thalamic regions processing input from arousal centres in the RAS of the midbrain. Studies of volatile anaesthetics have shown specific suppression of thalamic and midbrain reticular formation activity.

Finally, with regard to neurosurgical attempts to reduce severe intractable pain, the Montreal Group have noted that the multiple distributed activations in the pain system, as evidenced by neuroimaging, may explain why it is difficult to elicit (call up to consciousness) painful sensations by stimulating the brain cortex. It may also explain why local surgical lesions seldom lead to complete reduction of pain, though they may alter certain aspects of pain experience or behavioural reactions to pain.

The issue of consciousness and pain brings to the fore the question of mode of action of anaesthesia. It can be said at the outset that the way anaesthesia produces unconsciousness is not clearly answered. Animal studies with electrical recording from nerve cells suggest the basic effect of anaesthesia may be blocking of transmission of sensory inflow in the thalamus (see discussion in Chapter 11).

Sleep

The above discussion and analysis lead to a consideration of the results of neuroimaging of sleep. Sleep, of course, is essential for human wellbeing. Sleep deprivation is damaging, and insomnia is a cause of mental trauma. When a human is awake, the EEG detects bursts of electrical activity—about 8–12 per second called the alpha rhythm. When in a deep dreamless sleep, the EEG has slow, one to four per second waves of higher amplitude called the delta rhythm. *The REM (Rapid Eye Movement) sleep occupies about 25% of sleep time, and the EEG returns to a rapid wave form akin to the awake state. It is accompanied by a large loss of muscle tone, which,* inter alia, *stops the scenario of the dreams associated with REM being vigorously acted out.* Further—the distinguished French pioneer of sleep research Michel Jouvet (1992) of Lyon, arranged for his cats to sleep on little islands surrounded by water. The cats remained awake or went into slow wave sleep but when they went into REM sleep with relaxation of muscle tension the cats eventually slipped into the water and woke up. He found sustained long deprivation of REM sleep caused severely aberrant behaviour, hypersexuality, and death. REM sleep was vital to the existence of these cats.

REM sleep has its highest incidence in the fetus, and is very high in infancy and childhood.

The function of dreaming by the brain is not understood. Judging by the yelps dogs may emit when they are asleep, they may dream vividly. One theory is that with dreaming, instinctive patterns are coupled with new learned experience. The content of dreams very often involves basic instinctive elements such as fighting, feeding, escape, excretion, and sex, and rehearsing such patterns may be of value in enhancing specification of circuitry in the developing brain. Sleep deprivation has deleterious effects. It is the common experience of individuals with long periods of sleep deprivation that an extraordinary appetite for sleep can develop. It becomes an overpowering need to sleep. It is the imperious consciousness of a compelling need.

In terms of the choreography of the basic processes of arousal and sleep and the basic instinctive nature of need of sleep, neuroimaging has provided some fascinating insights. This is particularly when consideration of the results is coupled to other vegetative functions we have been analysing in relation to conscious processes.

With slow wave sleep, PET analysis by Pierre Maquet and colleagues (1997) in Belgium has shown deactivation of the dorsal pons and mesencephalon (midbrain), and also in both thalami and the basal ganglia. This deactivation may reflect the persistent decrease of firing rate of the diffuse ascending RAS, which causes the hyperpolarization effect (and thus reduced transmission) in the thalamic nuclei.

Also deactivation is seen in the orbital prefrontal cortex and both the Brodmann 24 and 32 areas of the anterior cingulate (see Fig. 9.1c) as well as in the precuneus and medial temporal lobe. The precuneus has been implicated in visual imagery and visual attention. This is evidently the opposite of the activations seen in many of these areas with thirst, breathlessness, and hunger. The lack of deactivation in these orbital–frontal–cortical regions with sleep deprivation may explain the serious disorganization of emotional behaviour in humans, including loss of adaptation through inadequate decision making.

By striking contrast, when REM sleep with dreaming supervenes, there is activation in the pontine tegmentum in the mesencephalic region, the left thalamus, in both amygdaloid complexes, the anterior cingulate and the right parietal operculum. At the same time bilateral deactivations occurred in the dorsolateral prefrontal cortex, as well as the posterior cingulate and precuneus. The picture is in general consonant with REM sleep being generated by neural groups in the mesopontine reticular formation, which activate thalamic nuclei and they 'turn on' the cortical mantle of the brain.

The Harvard-based investigator of dreams, Dr Alan Hobson (1988), has drawn a parallel between the mental scenarios—that is, the different type of processes that go on in the mind with dreams—and those that happen with insanity. In this regard, the striking deactivation of prefrontal lobe function with dreaming is perhaps consonant with the irrational character of dreams. There is no inhibitory control. In the context of dreams, the strong activation in anterior cingulate areas, which are also ignited by the conscious primal emotions may reflect anterior cingulate genesis of emotions associated with dreams. This could be as well as genesis of the characteristic autonomic effects (penile erection and cardiorespiratory changes) by descending transmission.

In terms of the overall pattern, it can be noted that the amygdaloid nuclei that are activated receive important projections from the dorsal pons and the intralaminar nuclei of the thalamus. The amygdala themselves have pathways down to the several brainstem nuclei, which could orchestrate the several conspicuous autonomic functions (e.g. circulatory, respiratory, and genital function—erections), which occur in REM sleep. The amygdala also send their most important cortical projections to the cingulate. Per Roland and his colleagues at the Royal Karolinska Institute in Stockholm have shown that with the transitions of relaxed wakefulness to high general attention by the brain, there is activation of the midbrain tegmentum and intralaminar nuclei of the thalamus (Fig. 10.5).

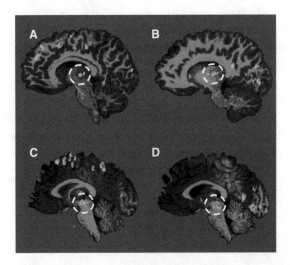

Figure 10.5 Areas in the brain activated by increased attentional demands. (A, B) Activation of the intralaminar thalamic nuclei. (C,D) Activation of the midbrain tegmentum (From Kinomura et al., Science, **271**: 512–515, 1996—with permission.) See also Colour Plate 6.

Micturition

Micturition, or the desire to pass urine, is one of the vegetative functions that intrudes into the stream of consciousness when the bladder fills to a certain threshold. If filling continues and is extreme, the sensation may change to one of considerable discomfort and eventually a sensation that is akin to severe pain. Normally, micturition gives rise to orderly voiding—emptying of the bladder—with a subjective sense mildly akin to gratification of other instinctive or vegetative functions.

Blok *et al.* (1997), of the University of Groningen, in the Netherlands, have made a pioneering neuroimaging study of micturition. It is set against a background of physiological studies of micturition on cats to which bank of knowledge Holstege and colleagues have contributed significantly.

The scans in humans were made under four conditions. The first was with a full bladder but withholding urine. The second was made 15 minutes later during successful micturition, and this stage breaks into two groups. Of their 17 subjects, 10 had successful micturition and passed an average of 567 ml of urine, whereas seven subjects failed at this point in time. They succeeded shortly afterwards and passed an average of 712 ml. The third scan was done 15 minutes after micturition with empty bladder, and a further scan was done 30 minutes after micturition.

A signal point from the data was that withholding urine caused a decreased blood flow (deactivation) in the right anterior cingulate (the Brodmann areas 24 and 32). This appeared to indicate that a general suppression of sensory input and motor output occurred to inhibit the sensation of a full bladder and the urge to void.

The act of successful micturition in the 10 subjects was associated with activation in the periaqueductal gray, the dorsal pontine tegmentum, and the front region of the hypothalamus. With the cortex, the significant activations were in the right inferior frontal gyrus and the right anterior cingulate gyrus (Brodmann areas 24 and 32) (Fig. 10.6).

The area activated in the dorsal pontine tegmentum was implicated in micturition control by animal experiments of Barrington in London in 1925. It is called the pontine micturition centre. It has cells that project down to the neurones in the sacral spinal cord, which control the bladder. The activation in the anterior hypothalamus (termed the preoptic area) is significant in that it has fibres projecting directly to the pontine micturition centre. The inferior frontal gyrus is involved in attention mechanisms. It may be involved in deciding whether micturition should take place.

The group of seven who were unable to micturate during the second scan showed an activation in the right ventral pons, an area which in the cat's brain had been implicated in the maintenance of continence. The unsuccessful subjects probably contracted their urethral sphincter involuntarily for emotional reasons, the signal going from this nucleus in the pons to neurones in the sacral cord which control the bladder sphincter.

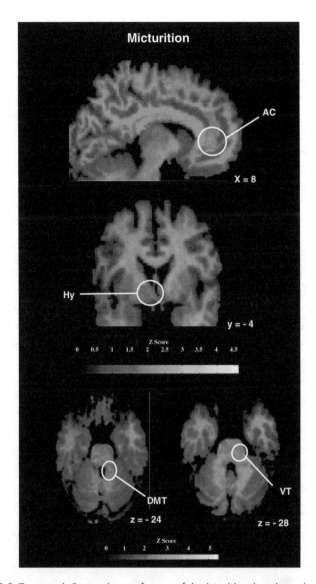

Figure 10.6 *Top panel*. Comparisons of successful micturition (passing urine) with voluntary withholding of urine. The anterior cingulate (AC) is activated. *Middle panel*. The same comparison also shows activation in the hypothalamus (Hy). *Bottom panel*. Left side shows activation in the right dorsal tegmentum with comparison of successful micturition with voluntary withholding of urine. Right side shows activation in the right ventral tegmentum (VT) region when unsuccessful micturition is compared with an empty bladder. (From Holstege *et al.*, *Brain*, **120**: 111–121, 1997.)

See also Colour Plate 11.

The authors draw attention to the striking fact that micturition control seems predominantly organized on the right side of the brain.

Jaak Panskeep (1998), as mentioned earlier, on referring to the feelings engendered by excessive bladder and rectal distension, notes that they become incredibly insistent, and fill the mind. He adds, the neural systems, which subserve such feelings, may be organized quite low in the brainstem level.

Stuart Derbyshire (2003) of Pittsburgh has made a survey of the literature dealing with visceral pain associated with rectal distension and other visceral mechanisms such as angina pectoris. His analysis includes comparison of rectal distension with oesophageal distension.

With rectal sensation caused by distension, the insula was activated bilaterally as was the orbitofrontal and prefrontal cortex, and the S_1 and S_2 somatosensory cortex.

With this gastrointestinal distension to a noxious degree, the thalamus, lenticular nucleus, caudate, and periaqueductal gray were activated, as well as the insula bilaterally, and Brodmann areas 39/40 (anterior parietal cortex) and the S_1 and S_2 regions responding to sensory inflow. Again, the anterior prefrontal cortex and the orbitofrontal cortex were activated, and it was of interest that angina pain activates these areas, as well as the periaqueductal gray and the thalamus.

The insula is central to these reactions in that sensory input and visceral nerve inflow converge on the insula where as Derbyshire says, sensory and emotive feelings may be integrated. The insula is part of a central circuitry that mediates affective responses to pain via its connections to the amygdala, and the fact that this structure projects to the perigenual cingulate cortex.

In general, oesophageal stimulation initiates more motor response and less activation of areas indicative of aversive reaction. The anterior insula was more activated by rectal aversive stimulation, whereas the oesophageal input was to the posterior insula.

A predominant finding of the studies was the activation of the cingulate regions of the brain. This involved the Brodmann areas 24, 32, 23, and 31 (see Fig. 9.1). The more anterior and ventral section of the medial surface of the cortex was more activated in lower intestinal distension than with oesophageal.

Sexual orgasm and ejaculation

The brain organization of this process of high biological importance in reproduction is being investigated by Professor Gert Holstege, Janniko Georgiades, Rudi Kortekas, and colleagues (2003). The experiments on males have been done in a positron emission tomography (PET) scanner with manual penile stimulation by a female partner, and scans associated with arousal and ejaculation are being compared. They note the co-ordinated action of male sexual organs and the floor of the pelvis, and the peculiarity relative to other motor acts, in that ejaculation is accompanied by orgasm.

The enquiry can be set against some very interesting earlier data on deep-seated brain stimulation in the human in 1972, associated with therapeutic procedures for epilepsy and severe mental illness carried out by Heath of Tulane University. Multiple electrodes were placed in the brain of two patients. In the case of the female epileptic patient, it was found that injection of acetylcholine or noradrenaline bilaterally into the septum (a region in front of the hypothalamus), made on 16 occasions on a weekly basis, gave mild euphoria, leading to a sexual motive state and followed by repeated orgasms.

Furthermore, when provided with a button device that allowed stimulation of the septal region at will, the patient stimulated this region 1000–1500 times in 3 hours, resulting in feelings of pleasure, alertness and warmth, and strong sexual arousal. Both patients displayed a similar EEG pattern when sexual orgasm occurred. The striking and consistent changes with recording from electrodes in nuclei deep in the brain were in the septal region with spikes and slow waves with superimposed fast activity. In one of the patients, recording electrodes showed changes also in the amygdala, thalamic nuclei, and in deep cerebellar nuclei. The efficacy of local deep stimulation in evoking highly organized neural activity involving change of consciousness in the human is clear.

Against this background, preliminary data of the Groningen group noted above are pointing to involvement of deep seated brain structures in the orgasmic process of humans.

Temperature control

With irradiation of animal life from the relatively stable aquatic environment of the rivers and swamps to dry land, new stresses on the stability of creatures arose. Analogous to the dangers of desiccation and the contemporaneous phylogenetic emergence of both a hormonal system of water conservation and of thirst, emergence of subjective mechanisms to keep body temperature constant carried high survival value. The primal emotion involving sensation of change of body temperature may arise from change of skin temperature or body core temperature. The spread into diverse econiches entailed animals evolving the capacity to obviate any deviation of body core temperature by a portfolio of physiological responses as, for example, the initiation of evaporative cooling. Furthermore, sensations from the skin and also body core involving severely unpleasant feelings will evoke intentional behaviour (e.g. burrowing or nest building) to counter the threat that may become extreme and threaten life.

Mechanisms emergent in poikilotherms (i.e. cold-blooded animals such as lizards and snakes) are that they seek and lie in the sun and their body temperature rises. Different mechanisms have been elaborated in homeotherms (so called warm-blooded animals). It might be predicted that the subjective sensations giving rise to intention to act will be organized in the phylogenetically ancient areas of the brain—the midbrain, hypothalamus, thalamus, and allocortex and transitional cortex.

As noted earlier, Craig proposes temperature control as a homeostatic emotion akin to pain. It is an affective motive with a feeling of pleasantness or unpleasantness according to the physiological context and is generative of behavioural mechanisms. This proposal, parallel to what is proposed here, is also consonant with William James' (1890) statement concerning life enhancing and pleasure, or objective injury and pain being explained by evolution having rendered subjective states effective in adapting animals to their environment.

At a reflex level of control, small changes of internal temperature of the body give reflex changes in skin circulation, sweating, or shivering, and in some species, non-shivering heat production. Dr John Johnson of San Antonio, Texas, a leading figure in this field of physiology, summarizes aspects of extant knowledge by pointing out that skin temperature acts in a so-called feed-forward way in so far as it can start regulatory responses before an error signal inside the body has indicated that internal temperature has changed. The response could start from the hypothalamus, where internal body temperature is sensed. Further, the set points or threshold internal temperature at which sweating or shivering is started can be determined by skin temperature. High skin temperature initiates sweating sooner, and low skin temperature initiates shivering sooner. Much of the data has been obtained from furred animals, and it is not sure how it might apply to humans.

Thus, a group from Australia and Texas have collaborated to study temperature regulation by PET imaging in Texas and by fMRI in Melbourne. (Dr Robin McAllen, Dr Michael Farrell, Dr Gary Egan, Dr Michael McKinley, Professor Graeme Jackson, and the author in Melbourne, and Dr John Johnson, Dr Jack Lancaster and Dr Peter Fox in San Antonio.). The idea was that increasing or decreasing skin temperature of the body would cause reactions of the brain cortex and basal brain regions reflecting temperature regulation responses.

The experiments were carried out on volunteers using a 'space suit' whereby water of desired temperature was circulated through a network of tubes in a garment covering torso and upper arms and legs. Skin temperature and body core temperature were measured. It was easy, and without causing any pain, to lower skin temperature. Then the brain was imaged and thereupon skin temperature was brought back to normal. The brain was imaged again when skin temperature was raised. This was continued so that body core temperature eventually rose also. In this circumstance, it was then feasible to lower skin temperature while body temperature was still elevated. Images were made over the course of the changes.

The major activity with cooling was bilateral activation of the sensory areas of the cortex as well as the insula and the anterior cingulate (Fig. 10.7). Heating involved the same areas but the expected activation of the hypothalamus was not decisive in the PET studies.

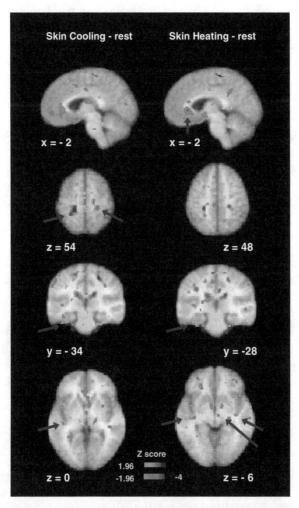

Figure 10.7 Activations and deactivations for the skin cooling (left column) and heating (right column) scans compared with the control scans for 12 subjects. The top row (x = −2) shows extensive deactivation in the left anterior cingulate; the second row (z = 54 and 48) shows extensive activation of areas responding to skin sensation; the third row (y = −34 and −28) shows left parahippocampal activation; and the bottom row (z = 0 and −6) shows insula and thalamus activation.

See also Colour Plate 12.

The anterior cingulate and primordial emotion

It is interesting that there is a remarkable commonality of areas activated in the anterior cingulate by primordial emotions of the vegetative states. Figure 10.8 prepared by Dr Mario Liotti and Dr Gary Egan is derived from our data on investigation of thirst and hunger for air, and also from the studies of Tatarinni and colleagues on hunger, Holstege's group of Groningen on micturition, Rainville and colleagues of Montreal on pain, and for comparison, Maquet and colleagues on REM sleep.

It is possible that these specific anterior cingulate activations during the respective vegetative states, in combination with other regions commonly activated with the specific primal emotion, represent a 'dynamic core' determinant of the conscious state. The other regions most commonly, though not consistently involved in every instance, are the insula, orbitofrontal cortex,

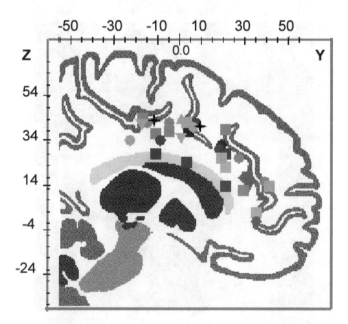

Figure 10.8 A diagram showing regions of the activations recorded in the anterior cingulate with positron emission tomography (PET) imaging of the brain during various primal emotions. Breathlessness (red squares); correlation with breathlessness (red circle). Thirst (green square); correlation with plasma sodium concentration (green circle). Hunger (orange square). Micturition and withholding urine (magenta). Pain—hot versus warm or neutral (blue). Rapid eye movement sleep (black star). The data are derived from papers on brain imaging under these specific states described in the text and included in the references. (See Liotti et al., Proceedings of the National Academy of Sciences USA, **99**: 2035–2040, 2001—with permission.)

See also Colour Plate 10.

claustrum, and parahippocampal and posterior cingulate gyri, as well as hypo-thalamus and periaqueductal gray. *Consistency would perhaps not be expected, as, presumptively, differing combinations would be involved in the specificity of the conscious state.* But it is possible, though not proven, that experiments like those of Robinson and Mishkin (1968) showing deliberative drinking deter-mined by electrical stimulus of the anterior cingulate indict this area as having a topographical (geographical) important role in the neural network subserv-ing thirst. It has been said, however, by Vogt that, in general terms, surprisingly little is known about the contribution of individual or structural aggregates of neurones of the cingulate cortex to function. This incomplete understanding remains one of the principal challenges for the next decade of research into this area of the brain.

It is presently transparently obvious that even if geographically specific cin-gulate aggregates are shown to have a role in the dynamic core of individual primal emotions it remains a great mystery how, if ascending input to the primitive cingulate cortex comes from the anterior wall of the third ventricle, thirst and intention to drink will occupy consciousness. Similarly, if from the hypothalamic nuclei, how hunger results, or from other hypothalamic areas how a specific craving for salt emerges. If ascending input is from the ventral front part of the medullary region and dorsal tegmental regions of the mid-brain—how it results in hunger for air, and if from Barringtons nucleus in the pons (dorsal medial pontine tegmentum) the desire to pass urine occupies the stream of consciousness. If the ascending input is via the spinothalamic tracts—pain is experienced. Presently, the actual basis of specificity is inexpli-cable. But it is possible that some cingulate aggregates are dedicated to par-ticular function and together with subcortical coalitions of nuclear groups are woven into the jointly sufficient and severally necessary elements of the dynamic core of the specific conscious state.

The REM activation sites in the cingulate are included for intrinsic interest and compari-son in so far as the genesis of REM sleep, as elucidated by Michel Jouvet (1992) and other distinguished researchers in this field, is from the midbrain, as is the case with arousal itself.

In an overview of the cingulate cortex and the influence epilepsy and lesions in that area have on human behaviour, as noted already, Devinsky *et al.* (1995) of the USA propose that the anterior cingulate has two divisions (see Fig. 9.5).

Overall, they see the anterior cingulate cortex playing a crucial part in initiation and motivation, and goal-directed behaviour. It is an agranular cortical region with extensive projections into motor systems, and is involved in many executive functions including those associated with affect. It is part of a larger ensemble engaged in these functions that include the amygdala, periaqueductal gray, ventral striatum (components of the motor system), orbitofrontal, and anterior insular cortices.

A comparable division of cingulate function into affect and cognition has been made in a review article by Bush *et al*. (2000) of the USA. It is highly pertinent in relation to what has been said in the foregoing to ask the question of what physiological and cognitive impairments follow lesions in the medial surface of either or both hemispheres in these cingulate regions. Broadly, effects of lesion in the region include, apathy, inattention, derangement of autonomic function (i.e. physiology of heart function and circulation, digestion, and other bodily functions not consciously directed), and akinetic mutism (an awake patient who can visually follow objects without any spontaneous motor or verbal responses), and emotional instability. Lesions resulting from arterial disease may bilaterally damage the anterior cingulate, but often involve other areas such as the supplementary motor area, and this is the context where akinetic mutism occurs. Damasio and Van Hoesen reported a case with a left-sided lesion of the cingulate and supplementary motor area.

The lady had no spontaneous speech or response to questions and no evident frustration. She recovered, and a month later commented that she did not talk because she had nothing to say—her mind was empty. The observations indicate profound behavioural disturbance and loss of experience of affect.

Elective recall to consciousness of emotional states: hierarchical organization

There is a clear ability to summon electively to consciousness some emotional states that may have involved distance receptor input in their initial genesis. In fact, the process of evocation by imagination is used in neuroimaging of states people usually consider when speaking of emotion. That is, hate, anger, happiness, sadness, fear, and disgust. Many elements, indeed much of the neural organization underpinning such emotional states, are genetically determined. This significantly dictates the specificity of the conscious content as well as the behavioural expression. This is nowhere more evident that in the evoked expressions of the face, whether human or animal, as was examined in his book *The Expression of Emotion in Man and Animals* by Charles Darwin. The threshold that must be passed in setting them in train may be influenced in some cases by internal states caused by hormonal secretion. That is, the organism is fired up and ready to react.

Antonio Damasio and colleagues (2000) at Iowa University have used the capacity of the brain to self-generate such emotional states to make neuroimaging studies. The subject is asked to recall and re-experience such emotional episodes. The point is that the neurophysiological organization of the brain permits this to be done. The emotional concomitants of the memory accessed or the scene imagined can represent a very powerful experience.

By significant contrast, it would seem that there is very limited capacity, if any, of the brain to be able to summon up to consciousness a full experience of the interoceptor generated sensations such as choking with breathlessness. Similarly there is limited capacity, at will, to bring to mind the full sensation of thirst. Stating this, I note that some people propose they can. It is questionable whether this does not really centre on imagining the experience of dry mouth which is not the same thing as thirst—though it can be a powerful sensation in the process as described by people lost in the desert. The same may be said for conjuring up in the mind the full experience of being hungry or suffering severe pain arising from the skin. One may approach it by the imagination of hitting ones thumb with a hammer. Also one might try to imagine pain from a viscus—you can feel you are getting towards it but not actually have the sensation. It is clear that there is probably large individual variation in capacity to imagine pain. However, the issue of being able to experience in the mind the sensation of a much distended bladder and the imperious desire to void urine seems to most people very difficult. In many ways the inability to experience pain in its full intensity by the imagination is probably a protective measure. The same might be said of sex in the sense that it is easy to conjure up in the mind all manner of circumstance associated with sexual activity and experience quite vividly the excitement involved, including changes in the body—particularly the genitalia. However, at the same time it is not possible to imagine a sexual orgasm as a full and intense experience—seemingly indistinguishable from the reality. In fact, it would be rather bad for the continuity of the species if this were easily feasible as a substitute for the reality. But, on the other hand, a sexual orgasm can be experienced in a dream. It bespeaks a dream having a different neurophysiological alliance with reality than an exuberant imagination has.

All these emotional states considered above involve extensive genetically preprogrammed neural systems, which clearly differ one from the other. For example, in the instance of fear arising from a sudden rearing of a snake in front of one, the visual stimulus will ignite neural networks in the occipital region which, together with frontal and cingulate regions will probably serve the perceptual categorization. The neurones will fire the amygdala, which the work of LeDoux and others have shown to be deeply implicated in the genesis of fear. The above-down process also will involve regions lower in the brain, particularly the periaqueductal gray area, the RAS, which subserve a very much heightened arousal. A train of various visceral reactions—quickening of the heart and respiration, and possibly an unpleasant feeling in the pit of the stomach, will occur.

The interoceptor driven side of the coin, orchestrated much lower in the brain, contrasts to these situational perceptions. Hunger for air arises in the base of the brain. The midbrain is also excited including parts of the periaqueductal gray, and also the dorsal tegmentum, the parabrachial nucleus, as is the hypothalamus. These in turn activate the thalamus and irradiating effects occur from there directly to the cingulate, and the insula areas of the limbic system of the brain. The arousal, which is set in train by the RAS is no doubt reinforced by traffic backdown from the limbic areas to the RAS. The tidal wave of emotion induced by these conjoint and contemporaneous excitations instanced is akin, in the very severe case, to the sense that one is about to die.

The point is that there are very different neurophysiological organizations involved in the above-down sequence of the distance receptor initiated emotions from those involved in the below-upwards events initiated by the interoceptors. This may in some way also underlie the capacities of being able electively to overrule to a greater or lesser extent the compulsions that the emotion generates in consciousness. It may also underlie the difference in capacity at will to electively summon the emotion to consciousness, and to experience it as a seemingly near reality.

Neuroimaging of the principal second level emotions: situational perception evoked by distance receptors

This categorization as a second level is arbitrary and relative. It is made purely to serve the purpose of delineating the emotions of, for example, anger and rage, fear, happiness, love, disgust, and sadness, from the primal emotions subserving homeostasis of the vegetative system (which similarly have major affective elements). The criterion of the dichotomy, as such, is that the usual evocation of emotions of the second level of the hierarchy is by distance receptor inflow (eye, ear, or nose), which sets in train either a direct reaction, or the reaction is secondary to the perception of a situation and the saliency of it.

The central fact of these emotions is that they are hard wired, and involve the basal areas—the arousal systems—just as the vegetative system emotions do. However, the perceptions setting them in train may be highly variable according to life experience.

Something approaching full psychic experience of the second level emotions can be achieved by thinking about situations and individuals. This has been a principal basis of neuroimaging. Further, there is the advantage that more than one emotion can be imagined in the one individual, so that comparison of states can be made in the single individual.

In the instance of anger and rage, it is known by electrically stimulating specific areas of the brain that the rage circuits run from the medial amygdala, through specific regions of the hypothalamus, down to the periaqueductal gray region of the midbrain. Jaak Panksepp (1998) points out that the precipitation of anger is entrained by environmental events, but these are not the only stimuli that can access the neural circuitry of rage—witness the inflammatory effects of imposed body restraint, or irritation of body surface. Panksepp notes that the subcortical anatomies and chemical transmitters for anger are similar in all mammals. Electrical stimulation of the same brain areas in humans has the same effects as in other species.

The onset of anger has wide physiological effects with increase in heart and respiratory rate, blood pressure, blood flow in the muscles, and rise in body temperature. It leads to a powerful impetus to strike. It is a major energizing force for violence with potential of survival value when there is an encounter with a hostile individual. Lesion studies have indicated a hierarchical organization of anger with the fulcrum being in the periaqueductal gray of the midbrain, which is the centre of inflow from above, as well as it being the genesis of outflow to the body systems that mediate the physiological response to the situation.

Antonio Damasio and colleagues (2000) have used PET imaging to study anger, and also fear, happiness, and sadness. The scan was done when their subjects recalled very strong personal emotional experience. For a separate scan they were asked to recall some personal episode that was neutral and without any emotional connotation. It was assumed that the elements of the recall mechanism *per se* would be common to both circumstances. Therefore, subtraction of the brain activity entrained by neutral episode from that where the actual emotion was evoked would reveal the changes specifically brought about by the emotion. That is, the neural processes concerned with image recall *per se* would be cancelled out. The PET imaging was done at the time the subjects felt the emotion. The success in engendering emotion was objectively assessed by showing increased skin conductance reflecting emotion induced sweating, as well as increased heart rate, and increased intensity of subjective sense of the emotion relative to neutral state. These physiological changes began before the full emotion was felt.

With fear, the circuitry subserving the emotion has been revealed by electrical stimulation in animals, and it extends from the central and lateral amygdala to traverse the anterior and medial hypothalamus, and extends to the periventricular system of the hypothalamus and midbrain down to the autonomic and behavioural systems in the brainstem. These latter cause the cardiovascular and other autonomic responses such as hair standing on end, or evacuation of bowel or bladder. As Panksepp points out, the behavioural evidence from electrical stimulation of the brain suggests all animals experience a powerful internal state of dread when the relevant areas are stimulated.

This is strongly supported by the fact that when these brain sites are stimulated in humans a powerful feeling of foreboding results with the fear being spoken of as being like some extremely unpleasant situation.

LeDoux in his book *The Emotional Brain* (1998) proposes a number of necessary conditions or concomitants for fear. Thus, you can't have a feeling of fear without aspects of the emotional experience being present in working memory. Further, you can't have a complete feeling of fear without activation of the amygdala because of the amygdala inputs to working memory, and to the arousal system. The inputs also determine the range of bodily responses that produce feedback contributing to the subjective sense. The arousal systems are essential in directing attention to the situation generating emotion. The feedback that occurs from bodily mechanisms set in motion by the fear are either experienced contemporaneously or remembered from previous experience. He notes also that you can have fear without being conscious of the eliciting stimulus, which may be processed unconsciously.

With regard to happiness and joy, Panksepp (1998) emphasizes the role of the play system—rough and tumble play. He says it establishes social structures and learning of social skills that can enhance reproductive success. Overall, play is a major genesis of happiness and joy. It expresses genetically wired systems in the brain. However, not a great deal is known about these underlying neural mechanisms.

> However, behavioural analysis, for example, in rats shows that rough and tumble play is very different from actual fighting. Study of the neuroanatomy of play and how it is compromised by lesions has emphasized somatosensory inflow, and the somatosensory cortex, and the role of thalamic nuclei in the motivation of play. Touch itself can provide great pleasure, particularly after separation, and can act to initiate play.

In Panksepp's experience, massive lesions of the cingulate cortex have little effect on play, but destruction of frontal areas as well as septal areas may increase play. This is interesting in the light of the neuroimaging studies of happiness to be recounted, which reveal rather massive deactivations of frontal areas.

With sadness, distress, and grief, a frequent element in the emotional state is that of separation, a state of loss, which may span from the sense of being left out like being discarded in a social situation, to the grief of permanent separation from a partner—or the death of one's child or life partner or friend. As well as the personal life situations that can determine these states, it is also clear that sadness and depression may arise from endogenous disorders within the brain because of abnormal biochemical and neural processes.

The results of experiments by Damasio and colleagues showed that activation and deactivation patterns in the brain differed qualitatively with each emotion. That is, there was specificity of the brain pattern coincident with the differing subjective state of the emotion.

Anger

The recall of the personal powerful episodes of anger had widespread effects in the brain (Fig. 10.9). Strong activations occurred in pons, midbrain, and hypothalamus, and the insula bilaterally. There were also activations in the anterior cingulate bilaterally and the left posterior cingulate and thalamus. Perhaps consonant with action elements inherent in anger (Panksepp's impetus to reach out and strike), there were strong activations bilaterally in the basal ganglia, lateral cerebellum, and the motor cortex.

Damasio and colleagues (2000) remark that the most visually salient feature of the study of the four emotions overall was the major deactivations in the neocortex. With anger, there were striking deactivations in the posterior cingulate, the secondary somatosensory cortex and the orbitofrontal cortex. There were also major deactivations in the lateral and medial prefrontal cortex. They also occurred in the parietal, occipital, and temporal cortex, including the hippocampus.

Fear

With fear, activation occurred in the midbrain, insula, and the secondary somatosensory cortex (Fig. 10.9). A very powerful activation occurred in the left parahippocampus, an interesting parallel to the fact that this was the site of maximum activation with thirst. It was activated also with food hunger. Strong activations occurred in the thalamus, the midline area of the cerebellum, and the motor area of the cortex. Similarly, with fear, there were widespread deactivations. A deactivation occurred in the hypothalamus and, interestingly, at a low level in the amygdala. Deactivations happened in the insula, and posterior cingulate, and the secondary somatosensory cortex. Again, powerful deactivations occurred in the orbitofrontal cortex, the lateral and medial frontal cortex, and the parieto-occipital and temporal cortical areas. These massive deactivations have a parallel to the same effect with combined hypercapnia and hunger for air. Whether it represents some turn off of selective but widespread cortical cognitive processes in a situation which is experienced subjectively as immediately life threatening is a consideration, though obviously conjectural.

A conspicuous fact in the neuroimaging in relation to physiological data noted earlier on circuitry subserving anger and fear was the absence of major activation of the amygdala. By way of possible explanation, Damasio (2000) notes that recalled stimulus of anger may be different from that entrained by visual input, which is undoubtedly the common physiological circumstance. Also, he suggests that data collection was made when the emotion was fully blown—in his view, the feeling phase as distinct from imaging when the emotion was being induced by a visual or auditory stimulus.

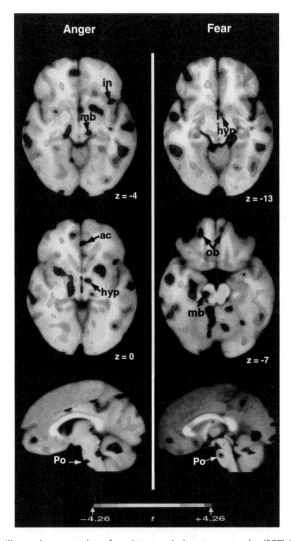

Figure 10.9 Illustrative examples of positron emission tomography (PET) images of self-generated anger and fear. The activations are in red (surrounded by yellow and green), and the deactivations in purple (surrounded by blue). *Left*. Anger has activated the midbrain (MB) and pons (Po), hypothalamus (hyp), and anterior cingulate (ac), and bilaterally deactivates the secondary sensory areas SII. *Right*. Fear. Activates the midbrain (mb), and deactivates the left SII, hypothalamus (hyp), and orbitofrontal cortex (ob). The deactivations of the orbitofrontal region is seen by the authors as a general feature of this study. They remark that the most visually salient features of the study was finding major deactivations in neocortical areas of both hemispheres (i.e. in frontal lobes and dorsolateral prefrontal cortices). (From A. Damasio *et al.*, *Nature Neuroscience*, **3**: 1049–1056, 2000—with kind permission.)

See also Colour Plate 13.

Happiness

Happiness recalled and experienced caused widespread activation in the brain. There were activated loci in the hypothalamus, amygdala, right insula, bilaterally in the anterior cingulate, and in the right posterior cingulate, as well as in the right secondary somatosensory cortex, and the parahippocampal gyrus (Fig. 10.10). Activation occurred in the basal ganglia, midline cerebellum, with again, deactivation in medial and lateral prefrontal, the temporal and parietal gyri.

Sadness

Figure 10.10 showed a generally similar pattern in terms of overall effect with activations in pons, midbrain, insula and anterior cingulate bilaterally, basal ganglia, thalamus, midline regions of the cerebellum and also in the orbitofrontal and basal forebrain. Massive deactivations occurred involving the posterior cingulate, the parietal, occipital and temporal gyri, as well as multiple foci in the frontal pole, its medial and lateral gyri, and the premotor area.

Extensive earlier studies of George and colleagues (1995) at the National Institutes of Health (USA) aimed at delineating the pattern of brain activation and deactivation associated with sadness in normal individuals. They showed activated bilateral limbic and paralimbic structures (the cingulate and medial prefrontal gyri and mesial temporal cortex—as well as brainstem, thalamus, and the caudate/putamen areas). By contrast, happiness caused widespread reduction in cortical blood flow especially in the right prefrontal and bilateral temporoparietal lobes—that is, effects in different areas of the brain. Mayberg, summarizing aspects of her studies at the Research Imaging Center in Texas in collaboration with Peter Fox, Stephan Brannan, and Mario Liotti, proposes that clinical depression reflects a failure of the co-ordinated interactions of a distributed network of limbic cortical pathways (Mayberg et al., 1999). That is, that dorsal neocortical blood flow decreases and ventral paralimbic increases characterize both sadness and depressive illness. Further, that concurrent inhibition of overactive paralimbic regions, and normalization of hypofunctioning dorsal cortical sites occur with remission of clinical depression. These reciprocal changes are proposed to be dependent upon a normal functioning of the rostral anterior cingulate as the pretreatment metabolism in this area is predictive of response to antidepressant treatment.

The general emphasis by Damasio of this particular study of comparison of four principal second level emotions in the same subjects was the distributed pattern of activations, and these involved loci in brain areas concerned also in homeostatic mechanisms, viscera, and musculoskeletal systems. The pattern of activation and deactivation within the regions of the insula, the secondary somatosensory cortex, and the cingulate are different for each emotion, and thus could be the basis of the different perceptual landscape with each emotion. The basal brain systems activated may contribute to physiological reaction, including those in the viscera.

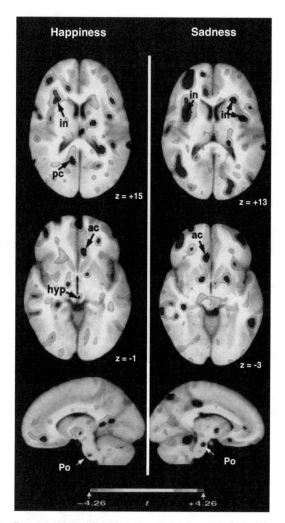

Figure 10.10 Illustrative examples of positron emission tomography (PET) images of self-generated emotion of (left) happiness and (right) sadness. The activations are in red (surrounded by yellow and green), and the deactivations in purple (surrounded by blue). Activations in happiness shown in these sections include insula = in, posterior cingulate = pc, hypothalamus = hyp, anterior cingulate = ac, and pons = Po. There is a deactivation in the pons, and in the frontal areas of the brain. With sadness, there was bilateral insula activation (= in), and both activation (anterior = ac) and deactivation (posterior) in the cingulate. There is an activation in the dorsal pons (Po). The authors note the pontine nuclei are unrelated to the reticular nuclei, and receive projections from the cingulate and insula, and send projections to the cerebellum, which may guide the cerebellum in modulating varied emotion action programs. (From A. Damasio *et al.*, *Nature Neuroscience*, **3**: 1049–1056, 2000—with kind permission.)

See also Colour Plate 14.

Part C

Higher cognition and emotion

Chapter 11

Anatomical structure and physiological functions subserving higher order consciousness

To place the examination of brain functions, primal emotion, and emotion generally in context, we consider here some theories of the higher order processes determining cognition and reasoning. These functions of the cortical mantle overlay as it were the brain processes subserving the primal emotions.

Vernon Mountcastle

Mountcastle (1980) of Johns Hopkins University has played a major part in emphasizing the columnar structure of the cortex and that this structure has functional implications. He suggests von Economo first described the vertical alignment of neurons in rows over all the cellular layers of the cortex, and that it was Lorente de No who first suggested a vertical mode of operation.

The primary area responding to sensory inflow from the body lies along the posterior border of the great central or Rolandic fissure (Fig. 10.4). Mountcastle's studies (1957) of anaesthetized cats showed that the basic functional unit of the somatosensory neocortex is a vertically oriented column or cylinder of cells. A column is capable of input–output function of considerable complexity. This is independent of the horizontal spread of activity in the gray matter, which is also a major feature of cortical function. The columnar organization of the cortex is exemplified also by the elegant studies of the visual cortex by the Nobel Laureates, Hubel and Wiesel (1997).

Considering the anatomical organization underlying the distributed systems or linked set of modules of several entities, Mountcastle proposed information flow through the system may follow a number of different pathways, and the dominance of one path or another is a dynamic, and a moment to moment aspect of the system. Similarly, the command loci of the system may at different times reside in different parts. At one moment a particular part has the most urgent information. The complex functions of the systems therefore are not controlled or localized in any of its parts.

The general concept of columnar organization does not preclude other systems—particularly those involved in general regulatory function engaging the neocortex in different ways. Mountcastle cites as an example, the nora-drenergic system arising from the locus coeruleus, a nuclear mass situated in the midbrain. It has, *inter alia*, been shown by Michel Jouvet (1992) of Lyon to be implicated in the organization of Rapid Eye Movement sleep. It projects to and can affect very widely distributed portions of the central nervous system including the entire neocortex.

We now look at some of the general ideas of how the higher cognitive functions of the brain are organized. That is, how the operations of topograph-ically (geographically) different regions of the brain are bound into a functional entity subserving higher order consciousness. This is a formidable problem. We will consider the ideas of some of the leading figures who have theorized and experimented to elucidate the issue. This will act to provide a broad picture of the more complex integrating features of higher brain function subserving con-sciousness. The primitive vegetative emotions when aroused will impinge upon this organization. The outcome of such a melange will operate to determine both situational evaluation and intention arising from the primordial emotion.

Changeux on the global neuronal workspace

Jean-Pierre Changeux of the Institute Pasteur and College de France is one of the great figures of contemporary neuroscience, and embraces also a great scholarship in philosophy and history. His book *Neuronal Man* (1985) is a classic. The later books *Mind, Matter and Mathematics* a discussion with the mathematician Alain Connes (Changeux and Connes, 1995), and *What Makes us Think*, a dialogue with the philosopher Paul Ricoeur traverse the impact of biological knowledge on questions such as whether mathematical laws exist as entities of the natural world independently of the human mind that formu-lates them. The affirmative view was taken by the mathematician and the con-trary view by Changeux who proposed mathematical laws are a construct of the mind. The book on discussion with the philosopher considered issues of human ethics. Changeux and his colleagues, Stanislas Dehaene from the Hopital Joliot-Curie, Orsay, and Michel Kerzberg of the Institute Pasteur, have proposed a neurophysiological model of a global neural workspace subserving *cognitive* tasks involving effort. This is distinct from a non-cognitive task which can be performed without effort. In this latter case well defined modules of cerebral systems specialized for sensory-motor processing are used.

The global neuronal workspace, the integrating element of the system as it were, is conceived as being composed of distributed and heavily intercon- nected neurons with long range axons. They can receive and send back hori- zontal projections to homologous neurons in other cortical areas. They can impinge on either excitatory or inhibitory neurons, and go across the corpus callosum connecting the two hemispheres of the brain. The connections mostly originate in the pyramidal cells of the second and third layer of the six layers of the neocortex. Some areas of the cortex such as the dorsolateral prefrontal (that is, upper and on the side of the frontal lobe) and the inferior parietal (the lower part of the lobe) are rich in this type of neuron. These neurones have strong reciprocal vertical connections with layer 5 of the cortex, and also with the thalamic nuclei, which allows *inter alia* one of many forms of direct access to the other main element of the concept—the processing networks. The first layer of the cortex involves a skein of connections over the cortical surface.

The second component of the idea involves a set of specialized and modular aggregates of neurones. They act essentially as processors for perception, memory, evaluation, attention, or motor function.

Those five major categories of these processors (Fig. 11.1) give mutual projec- tion to and from the integrating global workspace neurons.

Thus, of the five, as Changeux and colleagues (Dehaene *et al.*, 1998) see it, the *perceptual circuits* give the global workspace access to the present state of the external world. Temporal and parietal areas are particularly involved, including the areas subserving language comprehension. The *motor program- ming circuits* allow the content of the global workspace neurones to cause and guide future intentional behaviour. These circuits involve premotor cortex, posterior parietal cortex, supplementary motor area, basal ganglia, and the cerebellum and left inferior frontal lobe (Broca's area) controlling speech.

The *long-term memory circuits* contrive that the workspace has access to past events. This involves the hippocampal and parahippocampal areas. These will draw on other cortical areas according to the content of the memory. The *evaluation circuits* allow representations within the workspace to be associated at their simplest with positive or negative value. This means whether what is presently happening, as so accessed, is good or bad. These assessments are made by the orbitofrontal and anterior cingulate cortex, hypothalamus, amyg- dala, and ventral striatum.

Finally, the *attention circuits* allow the global workspace to mobilize its own circuits independently of the external world. As well as changing overt beha- viour, the actions may act to cause covert switches of attention so as to increase or decrease incoming signals from other processor neurone circuits.

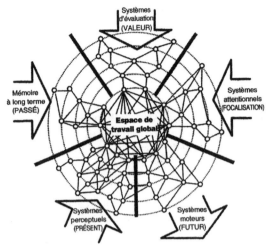

Figure 11.1 A representation of the Global Workspace and the major components of input and the output as envisaged by Dehaene *et al.* (1998). The systems feeding in to the Global Workspace (espace de travail global) are the present perceptions (PRESENT), the long-term memory (memoire á long term (PASSÉ)), the evaluation of what is perceived (VALEUR), and the focusing of attention (FOCALIZATION). The outflow from the workspace determining what happens is by the systems moteurs (FUTUR). (With kind permission from Jean Pierre Changeux, *L'homme de Verite*, published by Odile Jacob, Paris, 2002; and permission from the *Proceedings of the National Academy of Sciences USA*, **95**(24): 14529–14534, 1998.)

Other concepts inherent in the version of Changeux and colleagues of this hypothesis are:

1. These five processor networks project to the matrix of neurones composing the global neuronal workspace, but at any given time only a limited number of inputs effectively get access to it. This is achieved by a 'gating' process. That is, some inputs are admitted, others barred. Thus descending modulating flow from the workspace neurones to the processors either cut out or amplify the upward flows from processors.

2. It is proposed that a subset of the global neurones is activated in a sudden coherent and exclusive manner. However, only one such workspace modality can be active at any given time. This all or none 'invasion' differs from the peripheral processors. Here, due to local patterns of connections, several nodes with different formats can coexist. Thus one can smell, see, and hear an external object at the same time.

---

3. Changeux and colleagues suggest that neuroimaging studies have shown that automatic effortless processing, for example, characteristic of a thoroughly learned task can activate specialized processors in the cortex without requiring co-ordination by global workspace neuronal systems. The classic instance (of a learned task, apart from specially studied learnt and automated activity), is that of driving a motor vehicle along a familiar route to work while consciously working out reactions to the situations likely to arise during the day.

4. An early neuroimaging demonstration of learning becoming automated involved experiments by Per Roland and colleagues of the Royal Karolinska Institute in Stockholm. Seitz and Roland (1992) neuroimaged the learning of a task involving a complicated sequence of finger movements. Certain areas of the brain, sensory and motor areas of the cortex, which subserved the finger movements were activated at every stage. That is, during learning and when the task was eventually automated. However, it was observed that during the initial stage of learning some areas of the parietal and frontal cortex had an increased blood flow. However, this went away as the task was mastered and became automated. It was proposed that the change was due to the fact that the initial sensory feedback processing and the internal language activations required for learning disappeared when the subject was able to do it automatically.

5. Finally, and overall, the state of activation of workspace neurones is assumed to be under control of global vigilance signals. A primary instance would be from mesencephalic reticular neurones. These send the most powerful signals, which control major transitions between awake state (global workspace active) and that of slow-wave sleep (workspace inactive). At a lesser level, other graded inputs modulate the intensity of workspace activation, which is enhanced with the advent of novelty. It is damped by routine uninteresting environmental events. As an example of the neuro-chemical modulation of these processes, Changeux cites the recent study of Kilduff and Peyron (2000) showing that the neuropeptide hypocretin plays a critical role in causing discharge of the neurones of the locus coeruleus. This nucleus, noted earlier, is the site of noradrenaline excitation to the cortex. Absence of hypocretin in mice and dogs, which may be genetically caused, gives a behavioural disorder similar to narcolepsy in humans (sudden onset of sleep in day time).

Bernard Baars

Both Jean Pierre Changeux and colleagues, and also Francis Crick cite the ideas of the psychologist, Bernard Baars, of the Wright Institute in Berkeley, California. Baars wrote a book, *A Cognitive Theory of Consciousness* in 1988. It embodies the global workspace idea. Baars suggests the global workspace is something like the publicity organ of the central nervous system. He thinks of the brain as a vast collection of specialized automatic processors. Some are situated and organized within other processors. These processors can both compete and co-operate to gain access to the global workspace subserving consciousness. This enables them to send global messages to any other systems that are functionally relevant in the light of the extant circumstances. *The entire cortex is seen as a massively distributed system of specialized processes acting in parallel. Most of them are unconscious at any given moment.* The overview at present is that conscious processes are serial with one thing following another, as implied in James' term 'the stream of consciousness'. The conscious contents are broadcast to a collection of specialized unconscious processors. These in turn can compete and co-operate to gain subsequent access to the global neural workspace.

Overall, *the main entities in Baars' concept are these specialized unconscious processors, and the global workspace.* However, he also introduces the idea of *contexts.* Contexts are defined as stable working groups of specialized processors that have, over the course of time, gained a *privileged access* to the global workspace. *Thus unconscious contexts are a system that shapes conscious evaluation of actual experience without themselves reaching consciousness at the time.* They may reflect all manner of past experiences that shape emotional posture and attitude. They can include unconscious *expectations.* These may shape consciousness as experienced, but embody currently unconscious intentions that shape voluntary actions. Thus, if a set of preconceived notions are violated—i.e. surprised, then the expectations themselves may become rapidly accessible to consciousness. Overall, *contexts* can compete or co-operate to jointly constrain conscious contents. They are stable coalitions of specialized processors with privileged access to the global workspace.

It is interesting to consider one aspect of Baars' model. That is, contexts could be seen to reflect aspects of 'the caste of mind' of the individual. They are the conceptual knowledge, learning, imagery, and dogmas and beliefs modulating the perceptual process in the individual. A relevant illustration of context might be what Sir Wilfred Trotter in his book *Instincts of the Herd in Peace and War* (1922), termed the furniture that has been packed into the mind during the educational process. This, for example, may be the training to believe certain religious dogmas, and to see life through such a proscenium arch. Trotter remarks that

> The element of conflict in the normal life of all inhabitants of a civilized state is so familiar that no formal demonstration of its existence is necessary. In childhood the process has begun. The child receives from the herd the doctrines, let us say, that truthfulness is the most valuable of all the virtues, that honesty is the best policy, that to the religious man death has no terrors, and that there is in store a future life of perfect happiness and delight. And yet experience tells him with persistence that truthfulness as often as not brings him punishment, that his dishonest playfellow has as good if not a better time than he, that the religious man shrinks from death with as great a terror as the unbeliever, is as broken-hearted by bereavement, and as determined to continue his hold upon this imperfect life rather than trust himself to what he declares to be the certainty of future bliss. To the child, of course, his experience has but little suggestive force, and he is easily consoled by the perfunctory rationalizations offered him as explanations by his elders.'

Trotter goes on to say

> The mental unrest which we, with a certain cynicism, regard as normal to adolescence is evidence of the heavy handicap we lay upon the developing mind in forcing it to attempt to assimilate with experience the dicta of herd suggestion. Moreover, let us remember, to the adolescent experience is no longer the shadowy and easily

manipulable series of dreams which it usually is to the child. It has become touched with the warmth and reality of instinctive feeling. The primitive instincts are now fully developed and finding themselves balked at every turn by herd suggestion; indeed, even products of the latter are in conflict among themselves.

Trotter reflects on *the remarkable capacity of humans to espouse beliefs in the face of incontrovertible evidence to the contrary.*

Other contexts derived from group belief may be nationalistic and the world is replete with examples. Numerous other emotional postures and contexts may arise from past experience of the individual. Past experience may leave a portfolio of doubts, paranoid-like suspicions, and a sense of uncertainty, which will orient both appraisal of and attitude towards a new circumstance presented by the perceptual processors. Alternatively, the context might embody the training to evaluate events and situations on the basis of objectively verifiable scientific data. This needs a cogent discipline of analysis of cause and effect, amalgamated with scepticism and detachment from emotional influences.

Baars (1988), as an illustration of his ideas of the unconscious, suggests that a reader, as for example reading these words at this moment, is conscious of some aspects of the act of reading—the colour and texture of the page and perhaps the inner sound of these words being read. Similarly, one can become conscious of beliefs such as a belief in the existence of mathematics. However, it is clear that such beliefs do not consist of sensory qualities in the same way as the orange juice has taste, or the way elective recall to memory of corn flakes recreates the experience of a certain crunchy texture.

Descartes reflected on this matter in his sixth meditation.

> Moreover the ideas perceived in sensation were much more vivid and prominent, and, in their own way, more distinct than any I myself deliberately produced in my meditations . . . I saw the ideas I formed myself were less prominent than those I perceived in sensation, and mostly consisted of parts taken from sensation: I thus readily conceived myself that I had nothing in my intellect that I had not previously had in sensation.

Baars (1988) goes on to say, that in contrast to your conscious experience, one is probably not conscious of the feel of your chair at this instant. Nor is one conscious of a certain background taste in your mouth, or of the sound of music or talking in the background. You are not conscious of the complex syntactic processes needed to understand this phrase. Similarly, he says, one may not be conscious of one's intentions regarding a friend, or the complex processes in the semicircular canals of the ears that are keeping one orientated to gravity. Although one is not conscious of them, Baars suggests such unconscious events are being processed in the nervous system. In order to learn a new human skill, the acquisition involves a great deal of conscious processing.

Many different processors are involved. However, with time and thus practice, the task is relegated more and more to a single specialized processor. In reality, a 'distributed committee system' is supplanted by the development of a new expert system. The new skill becomes expert and automatic. We noted this in the case of the complicated learned finger movements studied by Per Roland.

Unconscious processes cannot be directly observed by ourselves. They can only be inferred from our own experience and observation of others. Baars points out that it was at the end of the nineteenth century that thinkers such as Pierre Javet and Sigmund Freud began to infer subconscious processes. This was on the basis of observable events such as posthypnotic suggestion, conversion hysteria, multiple personality, slips of the tongue, motivated forgetting, and like phenomena.

Baars' analysis considers short-term memory as being closely related to consciousness, but is not the same. He says it is practical and it is useful to consider consciousness as a kind of momentary working memory. Short-term memory then becomes a large current memory store that holds information slightly longer than consciousness does, and with more items.

However, there is also the issue of attention. In Baars' overview, attention involves control of the access to consciousness by reference to long- or short-term goals. The process may be volitional or automatic. It is clearly very sensitive to the significance of inflow, and such significance (Baars gives as an example the sound of one's own name) can be rehearsed to result in automatic priority of access.

Regarding the neurophysiological organization subserving the global workspace, Baars also emphasizes the anatomical and functional system in the brainstem and forebrain to have a crucial relationship with consciousness. Of course, central to this idea is the function of the reticular activating system (RAS)—being an elaboration of early ideas of Moruzzi and Magoun and Jasper. It receives input from all sensory and motor systems within the brain, and contributes crucially to interaction between these sources of information. It extends up from the midbrain to the thalamus, and the concept would include the diffuse thalamic projection system that has connections with all parts of the cortex (Fig. 11.2). Also, the cortical connections could be included so as to give an anatomical basis for what he would term the extended reticular–thalamic activating system (ERTAS).

The reticular formation subserves wakefulness, orienting response and focus of attention, and most of the central integrating processes of the brain. The fact is that damage to the brainstem tegmentum, including the parts of it—for example, the nucleus pontis oralis and cuneiform nucleus—may cause irreversible loss of consciousness. This bespeaks it having a central role

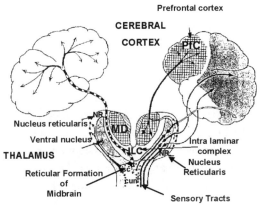

Figure 11.2 A diagrammatic model of a Global Workspace system with a coronal section (see Fig. 9.1b) through the midbrain and thalamus. The projections (arrows) between them and the cerebral cortex are shown. The shaded areas represent classical sensory pathways in the midbrain, the ventral nuclei of the thalamus, and the areas of the cortex (on the right side) with which these nuclei share projections. As the arrows indicate, the flow is both up and down. The cross-hatched areas designate the medial dorsal nucleus of the thalamus (MD) and the prefrontal cortex (PfC). The unshaded areas in the thalamus and midbrain constitute the reticular core responsible for the global activation of a tangential intracortical network via projections (dashed arrows) from the midbrain reticular formation (sc/cun) and intralaminar complex of the thalamus (ILC). The heart of this extended activation system is the nucleus reticularis of the thalamus (NR left and right side), which both 'gates' information to and from the cortex, and regulates rhythmic EEG patterns throughout the tangential network. (After Newman and Baars, *Concepts in Neuroscience*, **4**: 255–290, 1993—with permission.)

in the global workspace concept of conscious processes which is being advanced.

Pertinent to our general theme, this crucial anatomical structure, the RAS, controlling arousal in the mammals is a very ancient structure in vertebrate evolution. It is well developed in lampreys, sharks, fish, and reptiles. Figure 3.2 from Butler and Hodos (1996) shows the complex nuclear structure of the reticular system of the midbrain in the shark and in the rat. The rat is evidently more complex. As noted earlier, the neurones of the system have axons that bifurcate. The long branched processes may run both up and down the midbrain and connect widely. Butler and Hodos say that in all jawed vertebrates one can recognize without too much difficulty the main components of the system. These include the raphe group of the hindbrain, the parvocellular, magnocellular, and the gigantocellular groups of the medulla, the pontis caudalis and the pontis oralis group of the pons, and the locus coeruleus and the midbrain reticular formation.

The ERTAS, in Baars' eyes, underlies the broadcasting function of consciousness. During a specific moment, a selected perception 'processor' may supply particular contents. *The perception process bearing upon the outside world has a favoured relation with the conscious process.* Baars (1988) draws attention to the fact that cortical activity by itself does not become conscious. It must trigger the ERTAS in order to become conscious. Thus, a circulating flow of information between the reticular system and the cortex is required before sensory input becomes conscious. In this, the RAS may be a facilitator. But obviously the cortical mantle may determine the actual content of the conscious experience.

Baars notes that there is evidence from a number of neuroscientists, which would qualify aspects of the generality of the picture he is painting. This is, in particular, as it concerns the specificity of different parts of the RAS that have been discovered. In parallel to the concept that the cortical processes will determine the content of consciousness and the RAS may be the facilitator, the broad issues raised in Chapter 9 are highly relevant. This was the question of how activations in the anterior wall of the third ventricle gives rise to *the very specific* sensation of thirst, activation of the rostral ventral medullary nuclei gives rise to breathlessness, and activation of Barrington's nucleus in the dorsal tegmentum gives rise to the desire to pass urine. Possibly, as noted earlier, certain cortical areas, particularly cingulate regions, may be topographically dedicated to give these primordial sensations. However, it is also likely that the excitation of these particular conscious sensations depends equally on the specific midbrain and brainstem components, acting together with certain cortical areas to give the character of the conscious sensation evoked.

It is clear from the neuroimaging experiments on thirst as an illustrative instance earlier, that a particular conscious state may be associated with a distributed pattern of activations and deactivations in the brain. Given our present stage of knowledge of both central nervous function and thirst, some regional cortical changes that present in such a study of this specific physiological situation are in the category of likely suspects. Others are novel and perplexing. This is when we look at, say, all activations or deactivations, which are declared relevant and interesting above a significance threshold, i.e. a 'cut-off' point. A cut-off point is necessary to restrain what is sometimes an avalanche of data emerging from a neuroimaging study and is applied to avoid reporting false positives at an excessively high rate. It is arbitrary in so far as nuclei in the brainstem, which may be highly activated or deactivated, involve only a small mass of neurones. This small mass of neurones may not contrive a signal above the arbitrary cut-off level chosen because of its small size, and also the spatial resolution of the imaging system. However, the activations of these nuclei may be very important.

The seeming complexity of activations of different cortical sites that do turn up may reflect the manner in which a main process such as advent of thirst may ignite other areas in the brain, which subserve memory retrieval, or other thoughts and associations relevant to the state of occupancy of the stream of consciousness by the sense of thirst. However, there would need to be some commonality of activation of particular areas in the majority of individuals participating in a study in this regard for a particular area to show up. This is the standard situation with the subtraction method. The state of rest is prior to the procedure to induce thirst. It is compared with the actual images that are elicited by thirst. In general, a majority of the subjects in a study must have the same activation sites for the effect to be significant and thus show up.

In their analysis of the significance of activations and deactivations found in the course of neuroimaging a conscious state, Edelman and Tononi (2000) propose there is a 'dynamic core', and the components of it might be regarded as jointly sufficient and severally necessary for the conscious state. That is, they are central and essential. Other activation and deactivation areas can be reflective of particular aspects and circumstances of the situation evoking a conscious state, and idiosyncratic to the particular circumstances, but not necessarily part of the key elements subserving the particular conscious state.

The general conception of organization represented by the ERTAS has been elaborated in the writings of Newman (1997a, b) and of Baars, and the analyses they have written together (Newman and Baars, 1993; Baars and Newman, 1995). They emphasize that the stream of consciousness can only represent a tiny portion of the information flowing into and going on in the inside of our brains at any instant of time. A filtering process is required that must be very flexible and adaptively selective.

The organization involves the thalamus, as well as all information—auditory, visual, and somatosensory—passing through it. The thalamus is also the predominant source of internally generated activation of the cortex. Nearly all thalamocortical pathways pass through the nucleus reticularis of the thalamus on their way to the cortex, and this is true also of reciprocal pathways running from cortex to thalamus.

Architecturally the nucleus reticularis thalamus is ideally situated for central control and modulation of information flow between thalamus and cortex. It is suggested by a number of scientific leaders in the study of the thalamus enumerated by Newman that the nucleus reticularis represents a large array of gatelets controlling this information flow, a device that may determine selective attentions. However, pain, novelty, and danger, can all override the filtering effect exercised by the nucleus reticularis, which facet of organization is obviously of biological importance. Newman cites the idea of Gray on the content of consciousness. It is suggested that on a moment to moment basis, the content corresponds to the outputs of a comparator. This compares the current state of the creature's perceptual world with a predicted state. That is, whether perceptions differ from current expectations and involve novelty, need or potential threat, or involve cognitive schemes, purposes or plans. The predictable is the comparator which provides feedback to the ERTAS flagging whether present perceptions are familiar/expected or unexpected/novel.

The binding hypothesis

The key question, the overriding issue, is how do the contemporaneous activities in these various separate regions functionally bind in a unitary way to give the consciousness. This conundrum has been given the most consideration in the case of vision, where, as Francis Crick (1994) has pointed out, any object will have several characteristics (shape, movement, colour), *which are processed in different areas of the cortex* subserving the visual processes. Thus, seeing an object involves activity of neurones in different areas of the cortex. Furthermore, as well, an object may concurrently be smelt or heard, and thus more distant regions of the brain will be activated as well. Thus, the other sensory modalities are *bound* into the overall perception of a unity in consciousness—a sweet smelling flower.

Seemingly, a very important contribution to knowledge, as it concerns vision, was made independently by two German groups, Wolf Singer and colleagues (1999), and Reinhard Eckhorn and colleagues (1988). They found that neurones in two separate areas of the brain related to vision were firing at the same frequency of about 40 hertz (i.e. about 40 per second). This firing was in phase—not asynchronous. The point was that this firing was in response to the particular object. Both groups hypothesized that the phenomenon may be the basis of the binding underlying the conscious process. Various aspects of the evidence on this are described by Max Bennett of Sydney, in a book *The Idea of Consciousness* (1997), and, *inter alia*, he emphasizes the discovery that neurones in the thalamus, particular nuclei that Francis Crick (1984) has postulated as being generative of the searchlight of attention, also fire in the 40 hertz range. These may be causal of the 40 hertz oscillation in the neocortex.

In turn, these thalamic nuclei—the reticular nuclei—are greatly influenced by the brainstem nuclei including the parabrachial, the locus coeruleus, and the raphe nucleus. Koch and Crick suggested that the synchronized firing in the 40 hertz range of the various neural groups involved might be the basis of visual awareness.

In relation to the extant cornucopia of mysteries, it goes without saying that an overtone in the discussion of these exciting data is the emphasis by a number of the authors that *this important evidence of binding does not, however, tell how the binding gives rise to the conscious experience*. This is even if the neurophysiologically recorded data do reveal a crucial basis of co-ordination of dispersed neuronal masses involving complexity of connections to and from various cellular levels of the neocortex, including long axon connections across the midline. It may happen in a different way as Crick has noted. Jean Pierre Changeux, in his book *L'Homme de vérité* (2002) doubts the validity of the 40 hertz binding hypothesis.

Anaesthesia

It will occur to a reader who accepts the idea that some areas of the brain are critically involved in consciousness, that evidence in favour of such an idea might come from observing the effects of anaesthesia on the cerebral processes. That is, the study of events with transition from consciousness to unconsciousness and reawakening could be revealing of what cuts out and comes back in.

The question underlines the fact that knowledge of what happens with anaesthesia is relatively recent. Alkire and colleagues (2000) at the University of California, Irvine, imaged the brain during the induction of anaesthesia by two different volatile agents—halothane and isoflurane. A common basis of effect seemed to be indicated by the fact that the different anaesthetic agents affected the same brain regions. Anaesthesia caused an overall reduction of global metabolism of the brain but significant regional changes of brain metabolism were seen against this background. Particular regions so reduced included the anterior and ventrolateral nucleus of the thalamus, and the midbrain reticular system. Also areas in the inferior temporal gyrus, the medial frontal gyrus, the cuneus and the cerebellum had reduced metabolism. The authors interpret their data in the light of parallel findings on the physiology of sleep. They indict anaesthesia as causing a hyperpolarization block of thalamocortical neurones. By 'hyperpolarization' it is meant that the electrical charge on the neuronal membranes becomes larger, and therefore, the intensity of the signal to depolarize it and cause the neuron to fire becomes larger. That is, it becomes relatively resistant to transmitting a signal. The data were interpreted against the background of animal experiments by Angel of Sheffield, suggesting the primary action of anaesthetics may be the blocking of sensory information processing in the thalamus.

Fiset and colleagues (1999) of McGill University, Canada neuroimaged the brain changes with progressive induction of anaesthesia by intravenous administration of propofol. Again, reduction of global blood flow was observed but, on top of this, regional decreases were seen bilaterally in the thalamus, the cuneus and precuneus, and the posterior cingulate gyrus, which is itself closely functionally related to the precuneus. Regional decreases were also seen in the orbitofrontal and angular gyri. There was a close relation of functional change between the thalamus and the midbrain, underlining the role of the thalamus and the midbrain ascending RAS in the regulation of wakeful-ness. They suggest these changes attendant on anaesthesia involve the brain regions regulating arousal, performance of associative functions and autonomic control. That is, in the latter case blood pressure was decreased. In the article they wrote, they note the data of other workers, including Llinas and Plourde, which showed that 40 hertz thala-mic oscillations decrease in both natural sleep and during general anaesthesia. Fiset and colleagues discuss also the direct inhibitory effects of propofol on the cells of layers II, IV, V, and VI reported in Angel's (1991) earlier studies. They raise the question whether this is a direct effect of the anaesthetic, or the changes come about as a result of the decrease in the reticular activating-thalamus circuits, or the thalamocortical systems.

Other workers, Antognini and colleagues (1997) at the University of California, have neuroimaged subjects during mild and moderate isofluorane anaesthesia, and studied effects of touch stimulation. Tactile stimulation during the conscious state activated, as expected, the sensory I and sensory II areas in the post central gyrus area, but during low or moderate anaesthesia, these responses were abolished.

Overall, in relation to how anaesthetic agents have their effects on the function of the structures principally implicated, it appears they act by modifying the ionic channels of cells and the receptors linked with them.

Qualia

In the overview of present knowledge of consciousness, most writers return to the seeming impenetrable puzzle of qualia—the essential subjectivity of experience, which is intrinsically personal. That is, the blueness of the blue sea, the sweetness of a smell as the individual experiences them, are personal. There is limited capacity to convey by language what is felt, though it is assumed that other humans are having like sensations of, for example, colour—if they are not genetically compromised in their eye receptors in the case where the subject is colour blind.

An interesting neurophysiological approach to analysis of elements which are likely involved *as a hierarchical substratum to the emergence of a feeling as a result of a direct sensory experience* has been proposed by Rolls in his book *The Brain and Emotions* (1999). It concerns taste. Rolls has made extensive electro-physiological analysis of this sense. He remarks that in order to be conscious of the information in the form it is presented to the taste receptor and is first processed, the early processing stage must have access to the part of the brain necessary for consciousness. The data of Rolls and colleagues show that the neurones of the initial relay of taste sensation in the primary taste cortex (the frontal operculum and insula) are sharply tuned to taste stimuli. They do not alter in their responsiveness according to whether the animal is hungry or not. However, there is a secondary cortical taste area in the orbitofrontal cortex. The response of neurones in this area to taste stimuli in the monkey may decrease to zero if the monkey is fed to satiety with, for example, glucose.

However, if food with a different taste was presented and the monkey was prepared to eat it, the neurones responded to it. Thus, the response of these neurones was modulated by a state of hunger. It is experimentally established that the pleasantness of taste of food decreases when food is eaten to satiety, and this is commonplace as a human experience.

The output of these orbitofrontal neurones of the secondary area may impinge upon other neurones with food related responses, such as in the hypothalamus. The point Rolls develops is that it is only after several sequences of sensory information processing, that the sensory stimulus will be categorized. The quality of taste and its intensity is not affected by hunger. However, its pleasantness, and thus its rewarding quality is. Indeed, it may become unpleasant if the subject is fed on it to full satiety. An implication of the data is that for quality and intensity information about taste, we have to be conscious of what is represented in the primary taste cortex, and not of what is represented in the secondary taste cortex. But on the other hand, consciousness of the pleasantness of taste could not reflect what is represented in the primary taste cortex, but what is represented in the secondary taste cortex, or in other areas further on in the relay pathways where the object analysis systems project. This might involve the hippocampus, where memories could impinge on the consciousness of the sensation. At a further extreme, in higher cortical areas linguistic systems may operate to attempt to describe what is experienced.

Finally, in this chapter on higher order consciousness, it can be noted that Francis Crick and Christof Koch (2003) have recently elaborated their ideas on conscious processes. Their analysis places emphasis on what they term the 'penumbra' of neural correlates of consciousness (NCC). That is, whereas several coalitions of cells are involved in the consciousness process at any instant, and these include what Koch (2004) specifies as the NCC_e (the RAS and the intralaminar nuclei of the thalamus which are 'enabling' of consciousness) there are many other cell coalitions, which are operative, but are not contributing to consciousness. These could involve those subserving past associations of the NCC including intentions. The penumbrial excitations may become part of the NCC as the NCC shifts. The idea of the penumbra has a relation to what Baars has described as 'context' and also, perhaps, to what I have characterized as 'cast of mind'. This is the individual's cognitive and emotional posture, as dictated by past experience. Edelman suggests that, whereas the 'dynamic core' interacts mainly with itself, it is not totally cut off from non-conscious activities of the rest of the brain.

Apart from this overarching issue of qualia, and inherent subjectivity in the perceptive experience of, for example, the redness of an object, there is another highly challenging facet of the great mysteries, which is particularly pertinent to the thesis of this book. That is, how the characteristic subjective experience of an emotion arises. There may be a clear-cut specificity in the conscious sensation experienced. It specifies the character of behaviour set in train. This will be considered in Chapter 12.

Chapter 12

The biology of emotion

Poetry is emotion recollected in tranquility

Wordsworth—Preface to the *Lyrical Ballads*

Emotion is something of a real mystery. Introspectively, the individual knows the experience of the welling up from within of emotion, often nigh on uncontrollable. It may be in open conflict with what seems to be reason—a diagnosis seemingly more easily made with others than oneself. Or it may be the multifaceted pleasure of a perceived situation giving it a warmth and exuberance of beauty that makes it a culminating joy of life. The word is a portmanteau packed with diversity.

In my view, the existing diversity of views on emotion summarized below does not gainsay the major hypothesis of this book. *That is, the primordial emotions—the subjective element of the instinctive behaviour subserving control of the vegetative systems of the body—were the beginning of consciousness.*

The question of whether or not it is the best semantics to apply the term 'emotion' to the subjective components of the instincts subserving the vegetative systems does not determine the issue of whether such subjective (i.e. conscious) states, however termed, were or were not the first dawning of consciousness.

Examination of the biomedical literature, philosophical discourse, and lexicography, indicates that the many definitions of emotion which have been put forward reflect diverse viewpoints. In some cases, the criterion or criteria of definition employed would exclude phenomena that other definitions would embrace. Some feel it is extremely difficult to define. Everybody knows what it is until asked to define it. Also, central to discussion will be the issue of what is meant by terms such as 'feelings', 'motivation', and 'drive'.

Definition

The definition of primordial (a term Jean-Pierre Changeux suggested to me rather than 'primal') is evident from the use of the word in the text so far. *It is 'An imperious arousal compulsive of intention, which has emerged during evolution because it is apt for the survival of the organism'*. This definition assumes an essential genetic element. That is, there is vehement sensation conjoined with imperative compulsion to action. The definition is framed to embody the primal emotions where immediate survival is the issue. It is a conscious process.

I noted in the Introduction William James' (1890) view of the inexorable binding of emotion and instinct—a genetically determined structural relation. The definition I have used covers the case where the emotional state is fully expressed, but obviously much lesser degrees of evocation can exist where milder, low-level sensations would be beneath or only near the threshold of evocation of intention. Fitzsimons (1979) has addressed this in his book on thirst as mentioned earlier, when he compares the moderate sensation with what he terms the strong emotion when deprivation is severe.

In considering emotion it is clear that there is an extended hierarchy of types. These range from primal or primordial emotion subserving the instincts of the vegetative systems to the other extremity of emotional states that are determined by aesthetic appreciation or wonder. An example of the latter might be the awe of the grandeur of a scene, coupled with an intellectual appreciation of its significance. A case in point could be the sight of the Grand Canyon where the sheer overwhelming magnitude is melded to a knowledge that the geological history of the planet is before your eyes, and something stirs within. This sort of emotion comes from an intellectual process interacting with a visual impact.

A core element of Antonio Damasio's viewpoint

In this vein, Antonio Damasio remarks that human emotion is not just about sexual pleasures or fear of snakes. He instances the joys of listening to Bach, Mozart, or as he put it, the thick beauty of the words of Shakespeare. A pivotal element of his viewpoint is that the human impact of the causes of emotion 'depends on the feelings engendered by those emotions.' He sees 'feelings' as inwardly directed and private, whereas emotions are outwardly directed and public. 'The full and lasting impact of feelings requires consciousness because only along with the advent of a sense of self do feelings become known to the individual having them.'

This dichotomy, based on sense of self, proposed by Damasio, *inter alia*, would bring to the fore the question of how far down the phylogenetic tree some self-awareness is present. The possibility was discussed earlier in this book that it may go down very much further than operational definition by the 'mirror test' as shown in the great apes. In Panksepp's view it may go down to the first genesis of intention, which is subserved by the primordial motor systems of the periventricular gray and surrounding midbrain.

Damasio stresses there are states of consciousness where we may feel anxious, uncomfortable, pleased, or relaxed. Feeling did not begin then, but sometime before. 'Neither the feeling state nor emotion that led to it have been in consciousness, and yet they have been unfolding as biological processes.'

As a very distinguished clinician, Damasio centres the major thrust of his analyses on the greatest challenge—the human mind. A general aspect of his view and the dichotomy inherent in what he proposes, is encompassed in the statement—'Emotion was probably set in evolution before the dawn of consciousness and surfaces in each of us as a result of inducers we often do not recognize consciously: on the other hand, feelings perform their ultimate and long lasting effects in the theatre of the conscious mind', and also 'I suspect consciousness prevailed in evolution because knowing the feeling caused by emotions was so indispensible to the art of life.'

The overview on emotion, which is put forward in this book differs, in that the proposal is that *emotion itself represents the primordial event in the evolutionary emergence of consciousness in early animal life.* But, given the evolutionary elaboration of the brain, it is evident that even primal emotion may entrain both higher cognitive processes of thought, as well as basic body reactions such as autonomic responses (e.g. blood vessel and heart and respiratory changes). The latter may feedback and augment the emotional state. As a matter of fact, in relation to this latter process, it was believed by James and Lange that these autonomic and visceral sequelae were the actual cause of emotion, as distinct from the perceptions, or sensations of central origin being the cause.

However, as noted above, the emotion, entrained by basic brain processes, may then fire the whole amalgam of memory, associations, and reasoning. This then gives rise to complex feelings, and attitudes. One way of looking at this scenario would be in terms conceived by Baars. That is the emotion, and sequence of higher and personally idiosyncratic neural events it would set in train as reflected in feelings, would be determined by what Baars has called the *context* (see Chapter 11). Thus, in the particular individual, the cast of mind could reflect events of past life as well as reflecting immediately preceding events. Indubitably feelings are, as Damasio avers, a distinctive element of the conscious process. They might be distinguished from the raw emotion, but, as such, feelings involve a measure of cognitive elaboration of the contemporaneous conscious emotion. Anteceding events, including outcomes of previous behaviour will have dictated the context, the frame of mind, and thus, the feelings upon which the newly aroused emotion will impact and, therefore, be elaborated.

Considering the viewpoint I have taken that the term 'emotion' may designate a pyramidal hierarchy, the vegetative systems with the primordial or homeostatic emotions would be the base of a pyramid.

Dictionary definitions

Dictionaries have attributed a variety of meaning to the word 'emotion'. *The Oxford Dictionary* covering the English language, as they say from the time of the Saxon King, Alfred the Great, to the second half of the twentieth century, has defined emotion as 'disturbance of mind; mental sensation or state; instinctive feeling'. The OED definition also explicitly includes emotion as arising from bodily states. In psycho-analytic theory it is a state of tension associated with an instinctual drive. *Webster's Third New International Dictionary* notes its origin from the medieval French (mouvoir) and the sense of move out or move away. It declares it is 'an affective aspect of consciousness', and also defines it as 'A physiological departure from homeostasis that is subjectively experienced in strong feeling (as of love, hate, desire or fear) and manifests itself in neuromuscular, respiratory, cardiovascular, hormonal and other bodily changes preparatory to overt acts which may or may not be performed.'

Thus, it is clear that the element of intention and movement is incorporated in the meaning of the word, as is inherent from its origin in medieval French.

Going back to Damasio, he thinks the feeling of emotion provides the organism with a mental alert. Feelings amplify the impact of a given situation, enhance learning and increase the probability that comparable emotions can be anticipated.

As James (1890) cogently pointed out, blind instinct ceases to be blind after one enactment of the hardwired pattern—as thereafter cognition of consequences may be operative. The emotional states engendered by the first enactment of the instinctive pattern may irrevocably alter the evaluation processes thereafter. That is, the whole operation of higher central nervous processes involving insight and evaluation of events experienced will be operative in the future when the emotion is next set in train. The instinctive behaviour involving the intentions entrained by the emotion, may have had and still have high survival value. All this will represent a substratum of memory upon which any future evocation of the emotion will impact.

Thus, the overall state resulting is in a way idiosyncratic to the individual and personal history, though the circumstances that initiate the emotion and the propensity to respond are hardwired. Thus, contrasting the first experience of thirst with a later instance when, for example, the subject is lost in the desert, thirst may ignite a whole portfolio of cortical reactions. These could include self-castigation on the basis of stupidity of getting into the situation given past experience, of how it could have been avoided, or on the other hand, there may be also the reiterated imagination of a long draught of water as the individual becomes increasingly desiccated and the mouth is dry as a bone.

Edelman (1992) gives an overview of the issue in the one reference to emotion he makes in his book *Bright Air, Brilliant Fire*. He says, 'Feelings are part of the conscious state and are the processes that we associate with the notions of qualia as they relate to the self. They are *not* (author's italics) emotions, however, for emotions have strong cognitive components that mix feelings with willing and with judgements in an extraordinary complicated way. Emotions may be considered the most complex of mental states or processes in so far as they mix with all other processes (usually in a specific way, depending on the emotion)'.

This statement embodies the issue of intention ('willing') in emotion. It appears to separate feelings as being higher order processes than emotion with which they mix. The viewpoint expressed in this book is similar to that of Edelman in this respect.

Overall, it is clear that from the life experience (learning) and a person's disposition, innumerable different *situational perceptions* can initiate emotion—that is, the secondary emotions like love, anger, fear, hate, etc. The diversity is enormous in humans.

Ross Buck has put a psychologist's viewpoint in the book *Mind and Brain*, compiled with Joseph LeDoux and William Hirst in 1986. His proposal delineates a hierarchy of emotion, and stresses its relation to motivation—in my definition, the crucial amalgamation of sensation with intention.

The level termed 'Emotion I' by Buck is the most basic readout concerned with regulation of the internal environment of the body in ways that support life—homeostasis and adaptation of response to changes in the external environment. He instances maintenance of blood sugar (hunger), body temperature, water balance, and so on.

'Emotion II' is a higher level above the basic and the readout is accessible to other animals via sensory cues. It involves, *inter alia*, facial expressions, bodily movements, postures, gestures, and vocalizations—any behaviour that can be seen, heard, smelled, felt or even tasted, and will be indicative of intention to fight, flee, mate, etc. The emotion subserves social communication. It can be symbolically structured, the most advanced instance obviously being human language. 'Emotion' III in Buck's eyes deals with the interaction of emotion and cognition, and would seem to embrace the capacity of cognitive processes to initiate emotion, as, for example, sexual arousal.

Keith Oatley, Professor of Psychology at Toronto, and Jennifer Jenkins, in their book *Understanding Emotions* (1996), give as a definition of emotion 'A state usually caused by an event of importance to the subject. It typically includes, (a) a conscious mental state with recognizable quality of feeling and directed towards some object, (b) a bodily perturbation of some kind, (c) recognizable expression of the face, tone of voice and gesture, (d) a readiness for certain kinds of action.' This definition embodies the intentional element, and is evidently oriented to the human situation.

Edmund Rolls in his book *The Brain and Emotions* (1999) gives a definition of emotion that veers to the behaviourist viewpoint. As he puts it, the essence of his proposal is that emotions are states elicited by rewards and punishments. A reward is anything for which an animal will work. A punishment is anything that an animal will work to escape or avoid.

It is clear that many gradations can be recognized between what might be regarded as raw sensation (e.g. touch or pressure to the skin) and what has been defined here as primordial emotions, which are mainly interoceptor driven, and, therefore are primary and entrain a more complex conscious phenomenon embodying intention of high survival value. However, the distinction drawn is relative, as is also the case as noted earlier, between the primordial emotions, and those characterized by distance receptor activation, such as hate, rage, fear, love, etc. For purposes of classification, I have termed the latter secondary, being more complex in the sense of the mechanisms of activation and this often involves situational perception. They might also be termed 'classic' in the sense of being the circumstances to which the term is most frequently applied. On such an arbitrary view, the aesthetic emotions such as the delight and deep pleasure in being immersed in Bach would be tertiary—the apex of the pyramid.

Sensation

But coming now to the issue of sensation—as distinct from emotion. There are sensations arising from the integument of the body—touch of the skin, and itch. There are those arising from the special senses, such as taste, smell, hearing, and vision. There are visceral sensations such as nausea and vomiting, which are largely reflex through brainstem mechanisms. It is evident that an extreme psychic state can also initiate them, and if vomiting is preceded by nausea, considerable emotional distress may result. Of course, sensations arising from the specific sensors or receptors can in particular circumstances also entrain an emotion. The process of defecation, or urination, which has been instanced here, are essentially sensations associated with physiological function, and often without much conscious overtone. However, when they are impeded, thwarted, or when there is an endeavour consciously to suppress them, they can graduate from mere sensation to a conscious state involving anguish, distress, and something akin to pain. The simple events of sensation are elaborated by complex psychic processes. A simple illustration of this was in the neuroimaging experiment of withholding urine as distinct from simple voiding. It was seen that the anterior cingulate areas lit up in the withholding experiment.

The ideas of Panksepp on emotion

Jaak Panksepp of Bowling Green University in Ohio, like Joseph LeDoux of New York, has written extensively on the neurophysiology of emotion, and the analysis of emotional behaviour. Their books are great reservoirs of know-ledge. Noting the many attempts to define emotion, Panksepp (1998) suggests a distillation of the definitions might be such that when powerful waves of affect overwhelm our sense of ourselves in the world (a definition oriented to humans), we say we are experiencing an emotion. A weaker feeling might be characterized as a mood. He is explicit in saying that emotions are typically triggered by world events: they arise from experiences that thwart or stimulate our desires, and they establish coherent action plans for the organisms that are supported by adaptive physiological changes. Presumably he might not exclude a powerful desire *per se*, independently of whether it is thwarted or externally stimulated. Panksepp says that scholars down the ages have dis-agreed about emotion. They do not agree on the criteria to be used. As having a general definition that goes across species must include an analysis of brain systems, he suggests that the biological evidence indicates at least seven innate emotional systems are ingrained in the mammalian brain—namely, fear, anger, sorrow, anticipatory eagerness, play, sexual lust, and maternal nurturance.

He proposes there are many more affective feelings such as hunger, thirst, tiredness, illness, surprise, disgust, and others. In his eyes they need to be con-ceptualized in terms other than what he would call basic emotions. He then raises the issue of why he might not consider under the term 'emotion' feelings of hunger, thirst, pain, and tiredness (meaning, presumptively, an overwhelm-ing appetite for sleep). He thinks that the more traditional and cogent concep-tual reason is to exclude what he calls peripherally linked regulatory responses such as hunger and thirst from the category, and to instead call them motiva-tions. By peripherally linked, I suspect, he may mean the role of 'dry mouth' or 'hunger contractions' in contributing to the *centrally induced* sensation of thirst or hunger.

Panksepp's approach to defining emotions is said by him to be a focus on their adaptive central integrative functions, as opposed to general input and output characteristics. He says, apart from the basic psychological criterion, that emotional systems should generate subjective feelings that are affectively valenced, which is not easy.

Panksepp (1998) sees six objective neural specifications.

1. The circuits are genetically determined or hard-wired and respond unconditionally to stimuli arising from major life challenging circumstances.

2. The circuits organize diverse behaviours that have proved adaptive in the face of life challenging circumstances during evolutionary history of the species.

3. The activation of the circuits changes the sensitivities of sensory systems relevant to the behaviour to be aroused.

4. Neural activity of the emotional systems outlasts the precipitatory circumstances.

5. Emotive circuits can come under the conditional control of emotionally neutral environmental stimuli.

6. Emotive circuits have two-way interactions with brain mechanisms that elaborate higher decision determining processes and consciousness.

A classification based on six criteria reflects the difficulties, but if one were to follow it, it could be argued that salt appetite, thirst, and hunger, for example, would meet five criteria. They are hard-wired, generative of diverse behaviours adaptive to satiation, have changed end organ or sensory pathway sensibilities with deprivation (e.g. sensitivity of salt best taste fibres with sodium deficiency), the behaviours can be conditioned and interact with higher cognitive processes. A dichotomy does exist between the vegetative system dictated emotion and the classic distance receptor type in relation to neural activity outlasting the precipitating circumstances. With thirst, salt appetite, and hunger, the consummatory act of satiation can in a short time cause a precipitate and complete disappearance of the centrally induced appetitive state and associated cognitive processes. However, the chemical changes that generated the emotion may persist in the blood until the material ingested is absorbed. On the other hand, as Panksepp delineates, the central state of anger, or fear, may linger for a long time after the excitant cause has disappeared.

In relation to the six criteria or objective neural specifications, and the question of where sexual emotion would fall—whether like a vegetative system, or a 'true' emotion—Panksepp does note many reward objects that naturally satiate appetitive behaviours—food, water, and sex—have links to internal processes. Apropos of this, it is evident that consummatory behaviour with sex gives positive feedback leading to orgasm, which causes precipitate decline in desire and intention—just as with the consummatory act of satiation of thirst or hunger, or salt appetite.

The term 'motivation' would seem to have played an important part in the period when psychological science escaped from 'black box' behaviourism towards the issue of what actually made animals do things. The term had allowed discussion without too much reference to the idea of consciousness.

Panksepp (1998) says of the quasi-companion term 'drive', that it was used to indicate the incentive that the body need detection systems generated. However, he says such a broad abstract intervening variable cannot credibly be linked to unitary brain processes. He suggests the term is redundant for coherent explanation of behaviour. That is, deficiency states primarily facilitate response to specific external incentive stimuli.

Overall, he suggests that as we have to read the world around us on a periodic basis to sustain body equilibrium, we have brain mechanisms to generate various forms of distress (hunger pangs, thirst, coldness, etc.) when body resources deviate from equilibrium. We feel pleasure and relief when we undertake acts that correct distortion of the equilibrium state. *Apropos the use of the word 'emotion', it is without ambiguity that he notes affective states cannot be ignored if we wish to understand how body constancies are regulated by the brain.* The *Oxford Dictionary* defines 'affective' as 'pertaining to emotions: the opposite of intellectual.' The point of this is that his viewpoint, in my eyes, accords with the use of the term 'primal emotion' as applied to thirst, hunger for air, etc.

The nub of the matter is that the 'mouvoir' inherent in motivation would seem to place a prime emphasis on the action and intention element of the concept, whereas the popular connotation of the term 'emotion' is subjective. It is more coherent with the sensation as the prime mover. It sometimes has plenipotentiary power. The prime mover (cause) is sensation with intention as the effect.

However, Panksepp (1998) has suggested that the feelings of hunger, thirst, pain, and tiredness, should not be considered in the category of emotions. None the less he does note '. . . they have strong affective feelings'. The *Oxford Dictionary* defines 'affect' as emotion or desire, as influencing behaviour, and 'feeling' as an emotional state or reaction. Thus his term 'affective feelings' is close to defining these as emotions. However, he would term them 'motivations'.

Panksepp says it would be wasteful for evolution to have constructed separate search and approach systems for each bodily need. He suggests the most efficient system would be to have a generalized non-specific form of appetitive arousal, with various need-specific resource detection systems. This idea follows the overview of the ethologists as propounded earlier by Lorenz and Tinbergen. In *The Study of Instinct* (1951), Tinbergen cites Wallace Craig as using the term 'appetitive behaviour' to characterize the variable striving behaviour, which is plastic and purposeful. It leads to an external situation of particular character where an innate releasing mechanism then operates. This sets in train the consummatory act of satiation that is followed by a precipitate decline in arousal and interest. In the very first arousal of an instinct system, the random searching, exploratory, SEEKING behaviour proposed by W. Craig (1918), Lorenz (1950), Tinbergen (1951), and Panksepp (1998) could increase the probability of the creature by chance encountering a circumstance where the innate releasing mechanism, apt for the central arousal, is stimulated. Thereupon, a consummatory act occurs. Following this, learning may dominate the behaviour. That is, in the future, once distortion of internal conditions occurred, the conscious sensation would engender intention now directed at a quite specific goal. The animal would go directly to where memory indicated the desired material or situation—the goal—existed—witness the behaviour of the Mount Elgon elephants.

This scenario of a non-specific restlessness—proposes that the appetitive behavioural demeanour only veers to a consummatory act when the searching causes *chance* arrival at a circumstance that fires the *innate releasing mechanism*. However, I am not so sure from observation of sheep, who have their first ever experience of sodium deficiency as a result of profuse loss of high sodium content saliva from a parotid fistula, that the restlessness is entirely random. Though it is ensured that they never have experience of any contact with salt or salt solution hitherto, it is often observed that the behaviour of the naïve animal is to an extent orally directed. That is, we see licking, and chewing at metal bars of a cage even if all precautions are taken to ensure no dried saliva could have been present.

The case of a phosphate-deficient animal is interesting. If one makes a parotid fistula (Chapter 5) in, for example, a cow and replaces the sodium lost in the saliva, the fistula thereupon becomes a phosphate tap on the bloodstream. The behaviour seen as the blood phosphate level decreases and the state of phosphate deficiency progresses, appears to be a random chewing, nosing, and licking of objects. In a herd situation, phosphate-deficient creatures will chew one another's antler or horns—the restlessness being mouth directed. That is, the impingement on consciousness does not appear to be just random, but, to an extent, excitatory of mouth and olfactory exploration. The encounter with a bone represents the innate releasing mechanism for vigorous chewing. It appears on the experimental evidence from our studies that the innate releasing mechanism of specific bone chewing behaviour (phosphate appetite) is the odour cue coming from the dried medulla of a long bone. None the less, chewing and nosing behaviour is shown by experimentally phosphate-deficient animals before any encounter with a bone and sensory stimuli contingent on it is permitted.

In the same way, quasi-sexual behaviour may be exhibited by male puppies and young dogs involving copulatory movements with the clasping of the legs of unsuspecting immobile human males long before any encounter with a female conspecific has ever occurred. When such an encounter with a female conspecific happens there will be olfactory and visual innate releasing mechanisms to set in train the consummatory acts. The obvious predominant sexual arousal and quasi-mounting before any experience of meeting female dogs is not directed to any extent to exploratory chewing or drinking, but to unsuspecting legs of guests in the house, which is different and involves some rough specificity of orientation. That is, *it might be argued that appetitive behaviour is not entirely random*, searching, exploratory, and without any rough explicit direction imparted by the circumstances that have stirred consciousness.

What has gone before, which bears upon aspects of definition of emotion—what it is—leads to consideration of attempts by some authors to take an overview of what has been written in the field. Early on some, like English and English (1958), said that emotion was virtually impossible to define except in terms of conflicting theories. Plutchick in 1980 considered 27 definitions and echoed the same sentiment and noted most of the definitions did not refer to the subjective aspect of emotion. The idea of emotion as adaptive or self-preservation was mentioned infrequently.

Kleinginna and Kleinginna of Georgia Southern College in the USA, in 1981 considered some 92 definitions and nine sceptical statements. They categorized their definitions (see block panel for categories and examples). The block panel is representative of some of the definitions they cited. The differences in viewpoint are striking.

However, in relation to the use of the term 'motivation', which is akin to one arm (intention) of the amalgam I have designated as primordial emotion, Panksepp (1998) himself does emphasize the emotion as well as the motivation, both being associated with the vegetative behaviours. With thirst, and his recounting the Black Hole of Calcutta story, he notes the distress that such bodily imbalances create within the brain, and recounts *'the agony of thirst'* (author's italics). His stated need to understand 'the affective nature of hunger' affirms its emotional nature.

Panksepp (1998) states that when our rhythmic breathing is impaired by, for example, suffocation, 'A very powerful emotional state arises—giving a panic-like condition where the mind is rapidly filled with a precipitous anxiety'. In general, he sees several types of cognitive and emotional arousal occur in any strong motivational situation, and he draws attention to the incredibly insistent feelings of bladder or rectal distensions, which may fill the mind with nothing but the urge for relief. As noted earlier, he says, if we knew more about this we would probably understand more about consciousness than in most learned texts on the subject.

It is clear from Box 12.1 that many scientists recognize directly or implicitly the two components, sensation and intention, in their definition, e.g. William McDougall, Donald Hebb, Ross Buck, Jose Delgado Sidney Ochs, and Benjamin Wolman. Their definition would be consistent with the mode of use of the term primordial emotion here. The kernel of its use here may be seen as consonant with James. That is, it is the subjective component of instinctive behaviour and subserving the vegetative systems. It is interesting that Panksepp writes 'Sexuality lies at the fulcrum of our attempts to distinguish processes that psychologists have traditionally called motivations in which a bodily need is subserved by a behaviour, from those called "emotions" for which no bodily need is evident.' He goes on to say that obviously sex is not essential for survival of any individual member of the species but '. . . merely for the survival of the species itself.' He makes the distinction that sex is not just a peripheral body need but a brain need which has profound consequences for each species.

The distinction Panksepp (1998) is suggesting as a basis of delineating emotion from motivation is open to question (i.e. arbitrary) in so far as the

Box 12.1 **Panel of Definition of Emotion (Classified by Kleinginna and Kleinginna)**

Categories
Affective definitions

- William McDougall (1921): 'The emotional excitation of specific quality that is the affective aspect of the operation of any of the principal instincts may be called a primary emotion.'

- Donald Hebb (1966): 'Special state of arousal accompanied by mediating processes which tend to excite behaviour maintaining or modifying the present state of affairs.'

- Ross Buck (1976): 'Emotion is generally defined in terms of states of feeling. It is impossible to separate the activation and direction of behaviour, subjective feelings, and cognition.'

External stimuli definitions

- Robert Plutchik (1980): 'The characteristics of emotion may be summarized in the following way: 1. Emotions are generally aroused by external stimuli. 2. Emotional expression is typically directed toward the particular stimulus in the environment by which it has been aroused. 3. Emotions may be, but are not necessarily or usually activated by a physiological state. 4. There are no 'natural' objects in the environment (like food or water) toward which emotional expression is directed. 5. An emotional state is induced after an object is seen or evaluated, and not before.'

Physiological definition

- John Watson (1924): 'An emotion is an hereditary 'pattern-reaction' involving profound changes of the bodily mechanism as a whole, but particularly of the visceral and glandular systems.'

- Pavel Siminov (1970): 'From the physiological point of view, emotions constitute a special nervous mechanism which ensures the adaptive behaviour of higher living beings in situations which disrupt their habit systems, that is, when there is a lack of the information required for reaching a goal and satisfying a need.'

Emotional/expressive behaviour definitions

- Charles Darwin (1872): 'Actions of all kinds, if regularly accompanying any state of mind, are at once recognized as expressive. These may consist of movements of any part of the body, a wagging of a dog's tail, the shrugging of a man's shoulders, the erection of the hair, the exudation of perspiration, the state of capillary circulation, labored breathing, and the use of the vocal or other sound-producing instruments . . . That the chief expressive actions, exhibited by man and by lower animals, are now innate or inherited—that is, have not been learnt by the individual—is admitted by every one.'

Disruptive behaviour definitions

◆ Paul T. Young (1943): 'Emotion is an acute disturbance of the individual as a whole, psychological in origin, involving behaviour, conscious experience, and visceral functioning.'

Adaptive definitions

◆ Sandor Rado (1969): 'Emotion is the preparatory signal that prepares the organism for emergency behaviour. The goal of this behaviour is to restore the organism to safety.'

◆ Harvey A. Carr (1929): 'An emotion may thus be provisionally defined as a somatic readjustment which is instinctively aroused by a stimulating situation and which in turn promotes a more effective adaptive response to that situation.'

Multi-aspect definitions

◆ Jose M. Delgado (1973): 'Psychologists in general consider that emotions have two aspects: (1) The state of individual experience or feelings which may be analyzed by introspection and reported by verbal expression. (2) The expressive or behavioural aspect of emotions includes a variety of responses which affect (a) the motor system, (b) the autonomic system, and (c) the endocrine glands.'

◆ Benjamin B. Wolman (1973): 'Emotion. A complex reaction consisting of a physiological change from the homeostatic state, subjectively experienced as feeling and manifested in bodily changes which are preparatory to overt actions.'

◆ James P. Chaplin (1975): 'Emotions may be defined as an aroused state of the organism involving conscious, visceral, and behavioural changes. Emotions are therefore more intense than simple feelings, and involve the organism as a whole.'

◆ C.T. Morgan, R.A. King, and N.M. Robinson (1979): 'There is no concise definition, because an emotion is many things at once . . . the way we feel when we are emotional . . . the behavioural arousal . . . the physiological, or bodily basis . . . That emotions are expressed by language, facial expressions, and gestures . . . that . . . some emotions are very much like motive states in that they drive behaviour.'

- James V. McConnell (1980): 'Emotional experiences seem to have three rather distinct aspects: 1. The bodily changes associated with arousal and relaxation. 2. The emotional behaviour (such as fighting, loving or running away). 3. The subjective feelings that give a distinctive personal flavour to the emotion.'

Restrictive definitions

- Carl. G. Jung (1923): 'Feeling is also a kind of judging, differing, however, from an intellectual judgement, in that it does not aim at establishing an intellectual connection but is solely concerned with the setting up of a subjective criterion of acceptance or rejection.'

- Robert S. Woodworth (1938): 'Anyone will unhesitatingly classify as emotions: anger, fear, disgust, joy and sorrow; and as states of the organism: hunger, thirst, nausea, fatigue, drowsiness, intoxication. It is hard to find a valid distinction, unless it be that the typical emotion is directed toward the environment, whereas a state of the organism, such as hunger or fatigue, originates in intraorganic processes and has no direct relationship to the environment.'

- Paul T. Young (1961): 'In technical psychology, the term emotion refers to one kind of affective process and not to all. Among the varieties of affective processes are the following: Simple sensory feelings. Persistent organic feelings. Emotions are acutely disturbed affective processes which originate in a psychological situation and which are revealed by marked bodily changes in the glands and smooth muscles. Moods, Affect, Sentiments, Interests and aversions . . . Temperament.'

- M.S. Gazzaniga, D. Steen, and B.T. Volpe (1979): 'About the only distinction that can be drawn between motivation and emotion is that one usually thinks of motivation as arising from within the organism, often as a result of some biological need or hormonal influence. Emotion, on the other hand, is often thought to be a cognitive response initiated by an external stimulus. This is not a wholly valid distinction however . . . there are times when hunger is induced by seeing or smelling a particularly enticing food. Fear, too, can certainly come from an internal stimulus.'

Motivational definitions

♦ R. Leeper (1948): 'Emotional processes are one of the fundamental means of motivation in the higher animals—a kind of motivation which rests on relatively complex neural activities rather than primarily on definite chemical states or definite receptor states, as in the case of bodily drives or physiological motives such as hunger, thirst, toothache and craving for salt.'

♦ Sidney Ochs (1965): 'The visceral centres can be considered as the origin of appetitive drive states, and emotions considered as augmentation mechanisms intensifying the drives and leading to a satisfaction of those primary needs.'

♦ Peter M. Milner (1970): 'Motivational states that are not always accompanied by obvious external stimuli have names like "fear" and "anger". We call these states (which we are aware of mainly through introspection) "emotions".'

Sceptical statements

♦ Edmund Fantino (1973): 'In general, it appears that emotional behaviour is so complexly determined that a consistent characterization is at present elusive. It would appear, then, that little is gained by retaining the concept of emotion in psychology.'

distance receptor evoked emotions can have an obvious bodily need because fear causes either flight or freezing, either of which behaviour may ensure the immediate survival of the creature. The whole mechanism, with a central role of the amygdala, has clearly a high survival value for the individual and has been naturally selected because of this. Similarly, the overt display of anger and rage as a result of situational perception by an animal will be of immediate survival value by signalling the danger of fighting with it. Further, rage and anger can or will be an important immediate energizing and intensifying mechanism of high survival value in an encounter, though according to circumstances it may distort the judgement of the animal and get it killed.

The rational and emotion—suppression by act of will

Whereas the *relative* nature of the classification of emotion has been emphasized, there is some evidence of hierarchy in regard to the extent to which an emotion can be suppressed by an act of will. For example, when desiccation of the body in the heat becomes large, the sensation of thirst will fully occupy the stream of consciousness and an act of will can only extinguish it very temporarily, if at all. The subject may imagine aspects of drinking and assuaging the thirst, but overall the emotion is totalitarian. Coleridge's poem *The Ancient Mariner* depicts this well, as do actual accounts of survivors of shipwreck or being lost in the desert. Many of these accounts do also feature the terrible dryness of mouth and cracking of the mucous membranes and lips as a major sensation.

It is the same with the experience of breathlessness and the hunger for air associated with choking or suffocation. The emotion may be totalitarian and the ability to suppress it will be very limited. Similarly, there is a relatively limited capacity of will to obviate or dismiss from consciousness the urgent demand and sensation of pain caused by an overfilled bladder. It may increase to a plenipotentiary urgency above all other matters. The desire to sleep after protracted and enforced wakefulness can dominate any other element of the conscious stream. Torturers take advantage of sleep deprivation in extracting confessions. Severe visceral pain, as, for example, ureteric colic, would be another case in point. These statements are not intended to gainsay the fact that the attempt to make any general classification in a subject as complex as emotion will bring to attention exceptions that will be contradictory of the hierarchy proposed. Thus it is possible for trained persons, underwater swimmers, to hold their breath to the point where unconsciousness occurs. Similarly it is true that people go on a hunger strike and their will supervenes over the powerful desire to eat.

These examples represent the overall trend of emphasis—i.e. that these primal emotions have a measure of ascendancy, and in our hierarchical system they are not as easily suppressed by will. On the other hand, in the majority of cases within a structured society, anger, hate, and envy are suppressed or curbed to a sufficient degree that no violence ensues. However, obviously in some cases they may be so overpowering that people go to any other length to vent their antagonism and will kill.

Elective summoning to consciousness of emotion

There is a second criterion upon which some relative distinction can be made between the distance receptor evoked emotions and the interoceptor evoked primal emotions. This is the extent to which the emotional state may be generated as a conscious experience by an elective act of will in the absence of any exciting stimulus. The ability or inability to summon up the actual experience to consciousness may reflect basic differences in the organization of the brain subserving these differing emotional states.

We can set the issue of recalling emotions to consciousness in context by considering first the capacity to summon sensory processes to memory.

Hearing

It is clear-cut that the human brain can electively call to mind a particular piece of music and play it over in the present. Thus, a person may remember and play in his/her consciousness the C Major piano concerto of Mozart—No. 21. Neuroimaging studies have indicated that contemporaneous with the conscious experience of imagining of sound (the strong subjective experience of being able to imagine an auditory experience in the absence of real acoustic input), areas of the brain devoted to auditory experience light up while this elective pleasure is experienced. Indeed, nearly every region demonstrating excitation when actual sound was being perceived was also activated during the imagination of the music. Mainly, this was in the inferior temporal gyrus, but also in frontal and parietal lobes, the supplementary motor area and the midbrain. The involvement of the supplementary motor area may reflect that where a song is involved in the imagined task, activation of the supplementary motor area may indicate a covert vocalization component. Parenthetically, though it is hardly elective, the auditory areas of the brain in the temporal lobe light up when a schizophrenic hears voices.

Sight

Correspondingly, it is easy to summon to consciousness a particular scene, or the painting of a great artist, or the memory of a beautiful member of the human species, and experience vividly the picture in the mind. Per Roland (1987) of the Royal Karolinska Institute in Stockholm and Stephen Kosslyn (2000) of Harvard University, pioneered some of the neuroimaging studies showing that this volitional activity of summoning up a scene from memory melded with activity in the occipital lobe areas of the brain. These areas subserve the visual process. This imagination capacity is lost as a result of a lesion that affects a segment of the cortex normally involved in perception of that modality of visual inflow.

Smell

When we depart from vision and hearing and arrive at smelling, a different situation presents. Here there are some elements of uncertainty and controversy. Beyond debate, the sense of smell can be paramount in opening the vaults of memory—even childhood memories from decades ago. A particular smell will escort some long forgotten event into the stream of consciousness like a flood. Hitherto we probably may not have been able to summon the particular event to memory as an act of will. It had been forgotten. However, after the sense of smell caused such a memory evoking experience from very long ago, it may be possible easily thereafter to recover the memory of events. Perhaps the exemplar of this situation is the oft quoted account of Marcel Proust (1983) in 'Remembrances of Things Past'—the Swann's Way section of the book where he describes how the smell of the little madeleine cakes dunked in tisane tea brought back the flood of memory of experience decades before when as a schoolboy he visited his aunt, and she served him the madeleines and tisane tea at her home in Combray. Most people know this text, but in case a reader is not familiar, it is a remarkable description of evocation of memory.

> And soon, mechanically, dispirited after a dreary day with the prospect of a depressing morrow, I raised to my lips a spoonful of the tea in which I had soaked a morsel of the cake. No sooner has the warm liquid mixed with the crumbs touched my palate than a shudder ran through me and I stopped, intent upon the extraordinary thing that was happening to me. An exquisite pleasure had invaded my senses, something isolated, detached, with no suggestion of its origin.
>
> But when from a long distant past nothing subsists, after the people are dead, after the things are broken and scattered, taste and smell alone, more fragile but more enduring, more unsubstantial, more persistent, more faithful, remain poised for a long time, like souls remembering, waiting, hoping, amid the ruins of all the rest; and bear unflinchingly, in the tiny and almost impalpable drop of their essence, the vast structure of recollection.

The fact of this powerful capacity of smell, and perhaps also taste, to set in train memory is a different issue to the question of whether there can be the elective recall to memory of the actual sensation of smelling—summoning to consciousness and directly experiencing a specific smell. Can one just sit there and experience, because one wishes it, the perfume of roses, the bouquet of a particular wine, the smell of new mown grass, of faeces or what? And if it is claimed it can be done, explicitly can it be done without concurrent visualizing the thing that is imagined to be emitting the smell? For the author's part, I cannot convince myself I am able to do it even if I do also visualize a gardenia, a violet, a particular person with a particular perfume. One cannot grasp the phantom by the tail. Several friends, including eminent scientists who are attached to olfactory pleasures as wine connoisseurs, as bespoken by the fact of being able to identify often the wine in a masked bottle, say also they are unable to do it. It is an enlivening topic for dinner table debate. However, some people claim they can. Indeed, around a dinner table maybe 30–40% of people claim they can.

If someone tells you what goes on in their head, how can one know that it is reliable?

Dr Henkin, formerly of the National Institutes of Health (see Levy *et al.*, 1999a, b), has, with colleagues at Georgetown University, used functional nuclear magnetic resonance (fNMR) to image the brain activations that occur when particular odours are smelled. Then he has asked the subjects to imagine they are smelling such odours and not to visualize the objects emitting the odours.

It might be noted at the outset that the olfactory neurons have receptors exposed in the nose and the axons run to the olfactory bulb and then form into the olfactory tract on the same side. The axons from these run to the pyriform cortex and the anterior cortical nucleus of the amygdala and the anteriomedial part of the enterorhinal cortex, which is concerned with smell neurons. This primary olfactory cortex is situated near the junction of the frontal and temporal lobes and projections from it include those to the hippocampus, hypothalamus, insular cortex, and the orbitofrontal cortex where smell and taste input converge.

In the experiment of Henkin and colleagues the odours smelled were amylacetate and methone, which corresponded to the odour of banana and peppermint, respectively. The actual smelling of the odours caused activation of areas previously known to be associated with olfactory stimulation, including the orbitofrontal cortex (the undersurface of the frontal lobe, which is concave and lies on the orbital plate) and the enterorhinal cortex (Fig. 12.1), as well as regions within the frontal cortex including the cingulate gyrus.

Imagination of odours was tested in nine men and 12 women involving three coronal sections from anterior to posterior temporal regions. The activations in the brain were less than with actual smelling of the odours, and the activation with imaging the banana odour was less with women than with men. The regions of the brain activated by imagination were the same as with the actual odour. Changes, if any, in the occipital lobes subserving vision were not reported in these studies.

In patients with hypoosmia (impaired sense of smell), the neuroimaging response to odour was reduced. It was restored to normal by treatment with theophylline. Clinical studies have shown also that patients who have had various types of resection of the temporal lobe for seizures have impaired odour discrimination indicating that damage in the anterior temporal, probably mainly the piriform lobe, impairs smell. It has been found also that patients with early Alzheimer's disease have impaired smell sense, and all domains of olfactory discrimination are impaired in schizophrenia.

Lord Adrian (1969), Nobel Laureate of Cambridge, noted that it was very unusual for people to dream in smells, in contrast to the vivid visual imagery inherent in dreams. It is evident that the anatomical organization of the function of smell is very different from that of vision or hearing in that the initial relay from the

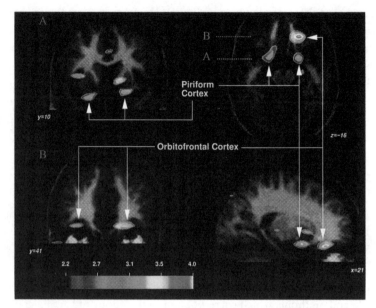

Figure 12.1 Neuroimages of a sensory process. The positron emission tomography (PET) images show activation (RED maximal) in the orbitofrontal and pyriform cortex when an odour was presented to one nostril only (the right). The effect was revealed by comparison with baseline when sniffing a non-odourous object. The top slice (right) shows activation on both sides in the pyriform cortex (at the junction of the temportal and frontal lobes), and also a large activation in the right orbitofrontal cortex. The orbitofrontal cortex was activated on both sides (see image at bottom left) but stronger activation on the right side. The bottom right sagittal images on the right side illustrated the position of the right orbitofrontal and pyriform activations. The orbitofrontal is part of the secondary olfactory radiation from the primary pyriform cortex. With kind permission of R.J. Zatorre and M. Jones Gotman, and Academic Press (a division of Harcourt Brace).

See also Colour Plate 3.

receptors situated on the nasal epithelium is to the rhinencephalon. This smell brain has a simpler structure of three layers of cells, rather than the six layers of cells of the neocortex (like the visual or hearing areas).

Taste

When it comes to taste, the situation may be intermediate between vision and auditory sensation on the one hand, and smell on the other. The question is whether there is some sense of actually being able to experience the taste of salt by an act of imagination, or likewise, extreme sour like a lemon, sweet, or bitter as with the tannin after-taste of a Bordeaux wine. Possibly a test of the validity of imagination that one was biting into a lemon and experiencing the sour taste would be whether one's rate of salivation rapidly increased. Evidently this occurs with a conditioned reflex, but this is initiated by a specific external stimulus.

Taste is transmitted to the brain from the sensors on the tongue by three cranial nerves—the facial which has the chorda tympani (VIIth) included in it, the glossopharyngeal (IXth) and the vagus (Xth). They arrive at the ventroposterior thalamus. The next relay is to the inferior area of the somatosensory cortex (post-central gyrus), and also to the frontal operculum and the front part of the insular. A secondary taste area is represented by the caudal lateral orbitofrontal cortex. Edmund Rolls of Oxford, has shown that the neurons there are finely tuned to specific tastes. Furthermore, that their firing may be modified according as to whether the animal is hungry or not. (Rolls 1999)

In neuroimaging studies, Kinomura and colleagues in Japan in 1994 showed that discrimination of saline from pure water was associated with activation in the thalamus, insular cortex, anterior cingulate gyrus, the parahippocampal and lingual gyrus, the caudate nucleus and the temporal gyrus. Functional activation studies by other workers have confirmed activation with tastants in the primary gustatory area in the anterior insula and frontal operculum.

Study of imagination of taste using functional nuclear magnetic resonance (fNMR) by the Washington University group have shown activations in the regions shown to be activated by actual tasting. The regions activated by memory of salt or of sweet on the other hand could not be differentiated.

Another interesting aspect of study of the smell and taste brain by neuroimaging was with patients who had persistent experiences of obnoxious tastes or smells in the absence of any external stimulus. The fNMR response to memory of the phantoms was activation in the taste and smell areas of the brain.

A further consideration of analysis of emotion and how Antonio Damasio sees it

In proposing this view that primordial emotion represents the first emergence of primary consciousness, it is obviously important to discuss further the imaginative book of Antonio Damasio, entitled *The Feeling of What Happens—body and emotion in the making of consciousness* (1999b). Damasio is a distinguished neurologist, working in Idaho, who brings to bear on the matter of consciousness a wide scholarship from clinical experience as well as a comparable breadth of outlook from learning in the arts and philosophy. He is primarily concerned with what happens in *Homo sapiens sapiens*, but his analysis emphasizes strongly that what he describes and categorizes has arisen in the course of evolution, and underlines the manner in which some conscious processes subserve the maintenance of homeostasis. He has a different view on the role of emotion in the hierarchy of organization of the brain to that expressed in this book, and therefore, implicitly a view of the first form of consciousness, which would differ from that set out here.

Damasio, in considering emotion, states that 'something like a sense of self was needed to make the signals that constitute the feeling of emotion known to the organism having the emotion'. In overcoming the obstacle of self, which meant from his viewpoint understanding its neural underpinning, he says it might help to understand the very different biological impact of three *distinct* (author's italics) although closely related phenomena: an emotion, the feeling of that emotion, and knowing that we have a feeling of that emotion.

In a section entitled 'The beginning of consciousness', he states that once he could envision how the brain might put together the patterns that stand for an object and those that stand for an organism, he began considering the mechanisms that the brain might use to represent the relationship between object and organism. He proposes that we become conscious when the organism's representation devices exhibit a specific kind of wordless knowledge—the knowledge that the organism's own state has been changed by an object. *The sense of self* in the act of knowing an object is an infusion of new knowledge continuously created within the brain as long as 'objects', actually present or recalled, interact with the organisms and cause it to change. The position of Brentano stated in 1874 that the basis of self-consciousness resides in the capacity of humans to recognize the differences between their own thoughts and sensory information coming from the outside world is clearly apposite to this idea.

Damasio says that in a curious way consciousness begins as a feeling of what happens when we see or hear or touch. He says, if phrased more precisely, it is a feeling which accompanies the making of any kind of image—auditory, visual, tactile, or visceral—within our living organisms. Organisms unequipped to generate core consciousness are condemned to making images of sight or sound or touch there and then, but cannot come to know that they did. He says, that from its most humble beginnings consciousness is knowledge, knowledge consciousness, no less interconnected than truth and beauty were for Keats.

In relation to what Damasio means by *core consciousness*, he says that it is the simplest kind that provides the organism with a sense of self about one moment—now—and about one place—here. The scope of core consciousness is here and now. Core consciousness does not illuminate the future, and the only past it vaguely lets us glimpse is that which occurred in the instant before. What Damasio is saying would seem very close to the emphasis that Crick and others whom Crick terms 'cognitive theoreticians' had put on short-term memory together with attention as crucial to consciousness. Damasio, as a dichotomy, says core consciousness has one single level of organization: it is stable across the lifetime of the organism: it is not exclusively human and it is not dependent on conventional memory, working memory, reasoning, or language. On the other hand, *extended consciousness* is a complex biological phenomenon, it has several levels of organization: and it evolves across the lifetime of the organism. Although present in some non-humans at simple levels, it only attains its highest reaches in humans. When it attains its human peak it is also enhanced by language.

Overall, the theory he proposes as the beginning of consciousness—the object and the organism—is essentially centred on 'distance receptor' input. It would seem to have an empathy in overview in this regard with the major Edelman thesis concerning 'perceptual categorization', which is analysis of distance receptor inflow and the making of a scene. However, in dealing with primary consciousness, Edelman does not appear to invoke self-awareness as seems implicit in the statements of Damasio.

Continuing to quote Damasio's views close to verbatim, he says the mention of the word 'emotion' usually calls to mind one of the six so-called primary or universal emotions: happiness, sadness, fear, anger, surprise, or disgust. The reader may note that he is using the term 'primary' as applied to what I have termed the secondary level or distance receptor evoked emotions. He is not referring to the primordial emotions in the instincts associated with the vegetative behavioural system. He says, thinking about primary emotion makes the discussion of the problem easier, but it is important to note that there are numerous other behaviours to which the label 'emotion' has been attached. They include, in his terminology, so-called secondary or social emotion, such as embarrassment, jealousy, guilt or pride, and what he calls background emotion, such as well-being or malaise, calm, or tension.

Having made a major distinction between emotions and feelings of emotion, respectively as the beginning and end of a progression, Damasio states, somewhat surprisingly in my view, that one may wonder about the relevance of discussing the biological role of emotions in a text devoted to the matter of consciousness.

Damasio says 'Emotions automatically provide organisms with survival oriented behaviours. In organisms equipped to sense emotions, that is to have feelings, emotions also have an impact on the mind, as they occur in the here and now. But in organisms equipped with consciousness, which is that they are capable of knowing they have feelings, another level of regulation exists. Consciousness allows feelings to be known, and thus promotes the impact of emotion internally, allows emotion to permeate the thought process through the agency of feeling . . . emotion is devoted to an organism's survival, and so is consciousness.' He remarks also that 'emotion was probably set in evolution before the dawn of consciousness'.

The general tenor or drift of this analysis based pivotally on the human situation and self-awareness would seem often a considerable separation between emotion and consciousness.

Self-evidently, from my viewpoint, I would agree there is a vast panorama of consciousness outside the consciousness of emotion, including the highest levels of reasoning, imagination, and creative ability. On the other hand, it is true also there is a great web of neural processes going on that do not reach consciousness. Attention is selective. *However, this does not seem to gainsay that emotion is an incontrovertible and very powerful facet of consciousness.* Exemplars include thirst and hunger for air, two primordial emotions not mentioned in Damasio's categorization above. Even if they are to be regarded as lower in the scale than, say, anger, it does not contradict the fact that they are very powerful conscious experiences with the potential for totalitarian domination as far as the flow of consciousness is concerned.

The nub of his view on this seems to be that consciousness only exists with a sense of self. The apparent self emerges as the feeling of a feeling. If this is correct, the viewpoint highlights the issue argued earlier in this book that self-awareness may go lower in the evolutionary scale than the self-awareness defined by 'mirror self recognition' (e.g. the instance of a trapped fox chewing off its own foot—Chapter 2). Mirror self-recognition is confined to humans and the higher apes. Darwin in his book *The Expression of Emotion in Man and Animals* (1965), seems in little doubt regarding the existence of emotions in animals, and that a powerful emotion may determine the subsequent cast of mind (functional structure) of an animal—its feelings on encountering a situation presaging the previous emotion provoking situation. Recall Miriam Rothschild's quip of taking your dog to the vet a second or third time.

If it is correct to make some dichotomy between an emotion and a feeling, this dichotomy is perhaps largely, though not exclusively, a human phenomenon directly contingent on a highly developed self-awareness. There is little doubt that a primal emotion may be overlaid in a self-aware organism by a portfolio of feelings, apprehension, and disquiet—and sometimes fear in the light of past experience.

Dolan (2002), of the renowned Wellcome Department of Imaging Neuroscience at Queens Square, London, has written in *Science* on emotion. He makes the important general point, which would be the experience of most doctors. A lack of emotional equilibrium underpins most human unhappiness and is a common denominator in psychiatric practice from neuroses to psychoses. He emphasizes the global effects of emotions as distinct from other psychological states on all aspects of cognition. He emphasizes their role in directing attention. He also notes that in situations where higher cortical function associated with vision is impaired because of a lesion, there is evidence that preconscious processing of emotional stimuli (pre-attentive processing) can give enhanced stimulus detection—i.e. perception. He also stresses the role of the amygdala in emotional memory.

Like Damasio, Dolan (2002) makes a distinction between emotion and feeling. He says 'Feelings are defined as *mental representations of physiological changes* (author's italics) that characterize and are consequent upon processing emotion—eliciting objects or states.' This seems rather close to using the term 'feelings' in a sense close to James' original definition in 1884 of emotion, namely '*My theory . . . . Is that the bodily changes follow directly the perception of the exciting fact, and that our feeling of the same changes as they occur is the emotion.* This particular idea of origin of emotion is not now usually accepted. However, Dolan's idea, as he says, does assign an important role to afferent feedback to the brain—sensory and neurochemical—arising from changes in bodily state caused by the emotion. As such, they contribute to an amalgam of elements associated with the primary central genesis.

To me it seems that physiological feedback will be one of the components of the emotional state. The emotional state generated is primarily in the telencephalon, i.e. centrally. The elaboration of the emotion to what is termed 'feelings' involves essentially cognitive processes therein. This can embody a complex of situational perception, influenced by, in particular, memory, with expectation of consequences and sense of past excitement, and present apprehension. Without doubt, as indicated, the emotion can be amplified by feedback of visceral sensation set in train by the initial perception. Further, there may be superimposed intellectual appraisal of the weight of various options that might be exercised. Dolan (2002) notes that the role of afferent feedback is underlined by the fact that patients with pure autonomic failure—a breakdown of peripheral autonomic regulation—have a subtle blunting of emotional experience.

Concluding remarks on emotion

In my view, processes generating emotion reflect an integrative and genetically determined coherent neural organization with a significant part of it in the telencephalon—a distributed but functional unified system. As hypothesized, consciousness probably emerged phylogenetically with elaboration of connections of the mesencephalon and diencephalon with the developing telencephalon.

The perspective envisaged is that, for example, early in evolution the sensing of biochemical changes—rise in blood sodium concentration—by structures in the hypothalamus, did cause antidiuretic hormone release, which in turn causes water retention. This physiologically apt response occurs at a level below consciousness. It is a homeostatic process. However, it is true also that in higher animals it can be *accessed and modified by conscious processes.* Fear and apprehension, i.e. high-level emotional processes, can cause antidiuretic hormone release in the water replete mammal. In like vein, increase in sodium concentration in the blood in bony fishes will cause increased drinking, which involves increased abstraction of water from sea water. This response is probably reflex. However, later in evolution water was not part of the immediate milieu of existence of most vertebrate species. An automated swallowing response could no longer correct chemical distortion, which occurred when migration on to dry land happened. The situation had changed dramatically. *Thereupon the saliency of the sensing of body desiccation by hypothalamic sensors took on a quite different role.* Certainly apt antidiuretic hormone secretion continued to occur. However, the cardinal biological relevance of the sensing was inextricably linked to the fact that thirst evolved. This led to the impetus, the intention to seek, find and drink water. That is consciousness emerged with further development rostrally of the brain. Then specific telencephalic structures, some of which, would seem to have been identified in our neuroimaging experiments, responded to upwards flow of stimuli from the sodium (osmotic) sensors in the hypothalamus. Similarly, upward flow would come from the arousal mechanisms of the midbrain—thalamic reticular activating system. The cerebral neuroanatomy that developed, including allocortex and transitional cortex, became part of the distributed system subserving emergence of thirst. Consciousness of thirst emerged as an interoceptor (i.e. internal sensor) driven phenomenon. The hypothalamic–midbrain mechanisms for sensing changes of solute concentration became spectacularly more pertinent for survival, as were the apt intentions subserving this end. This type of development was true generally in the vegetative systems whether what was sensed was change in salt concentration of blood, rise in arterial carbon dioxide concentration, rise or fall in blood temperature, or fall in blood glucose concentration with hunger initiating a hunt for prey.

It is evident that Damasio also emphasizes a hierarchical structure of consciousness. This is reflective of both differences in neurophysiological organizations and the reality of evolutionary history leading to the peak of the hierarchy of emotions as say, the attendant feeling engendered by listening to Bach. Such a dissection of elements in the higher realms of conscious processes in humans is stimulating, imaginative, and evocative. However, it is also true that the very quintessence of emotion is exemplified when there is a totalitarian invasion of the stream of consciousness by, for example, primordial hunger for air when the air supply is cut off.

In my view the word is explicitly appropriate, as the Oxford Dictionary, and also William James (1890) aver, to the conscious perception of change in bodily states, which I have been concerned with analysing and discussing, as well as those of rage, fear, and so on. Damasio suggests the evidence is that most, if not all, emotional responses are a result of a long history of evolutionary fine tuning—bioregulatory devices with which we come equipped in order to survive.

Thus, I would propose the emotions of the vegetative physiological regulations are the most basic, whereas those proposed by Damasio as primary—namely, happiness, sadness, fear, anger, surprise, and disgust are different. They are rather of a higher order in the sense of being distance receptor evoked, and most often a situational perception underlies firing these hard-wired systems. *However, both the primordial and distance receptor emotions are hardwired organizations and the classification is a matter of relativity. To an extent the distance receptor ones act from above down, whereas the interoceptor driven ones act from below—upwards.* This arbitrariness (that is ambiguity in definition) is illustrated by the evidence that powerful sexual drive, an emotion arising from the vegetative system, may be interoceptor or exteroceptor driven, and may be volitionarily controlled, or may not—analogous to explosive anger. Damasio also notes the fact of arbitrariness of definition of emotion. In his chapter footnotes he says that deciding what constitutes an emotion is not an easy task, and once you survey the whole range of possible phenomena one does wonder if any sensible definition of emotion can be formulated, and if a single term remains useful to describe all these states. He notes that others have struggled with the problem and concluded it is hopeless.

At the one hand there is Damasio's view that emotions were initially beneath the level of consciousness and became evident when the phylogenetic emergence of sense of self—self-awareness—allowed feelings. However, he does also say that 'At their most basic, emotions are part of homeostatic regulation and are poised to avoid loss of integrity that is a harbinger of death, or death itself, as well as to endorse a source of energy, shelter, or sex'. On the other hand, *an alternative view to his first statement is that the evolution of the genetically programmed response systems—the instincts of the vegetative systems with high survival value—involved subjectivity, which are the primordial emotions.*

Indeed, the last word on classification might be left to James (1890):

> If one should seek to name each particular one of them of which the human heart is the seat, it is plain the limit to their number would be in the introspective vocabulary of the seeker, each race of men having found names for some shade of feeling which other races have left undiscriminated . . . The reader can then class emotions as he will, as sad or joyous, sthenic or asthenic, natural or acquired, inspired by animate or inanimate things, formal or material, sensuous or ideal, direct or reflective, egoistic or non-egoistic, retrospective, prospective or immediate, organismally or environmentally initiated or what more besides. Each of those proposed divisions has its merits, and each one brings together some emotions which the others keep apart.

The position I have taken in this book is coherent with William James' view advanced a century ago on the inexorable binding of emotion and instinct— 'They shade imperceptibly into each other.'

Summary

In summary, emotions are a mystery. To repeat what Edelman said

> Feelings are part of the conscious state. But they are not emotions. Emotions have strong cognitive components that mix feelings with willing, and also judgements in an extraordinarily complex way. Emotions may be considered the most complex mental states in so far as they mix with all other processes, and in a very specific way depending on the emotion.

Obviously they vary in intensity according to circumstances, and may well up to give a totalitarian occupancy of consciousness. They may be overpowering and submerge any will or rationality hitherto operative.

They include the subjective component of genetically programmed neural systems of high survival value—the vegetative regulatory systems, as well as the distance receptor activated neural circuits subserving anger, fear, etc.

Thus, they are conserved in the phylogenetic tree. Neurophysiological investigation has shown that the same groups of neurons—nuclei—operate similarly lower down the phylogenetic tree.

The different types of emotion are mediated by separate neural systems, and this is evident in neuroimaging studies. However, there are clearly neural centres that are strong components in several emotions, as, for example, the insula and cingulate gyrus. In the human, at least, where we have introspective abilities, it is clear that there are limitations to the ability to electively summon to consciousness the experience of a particular emotion. It is quite different to the ability of the will to bring to consciousness a particular scene or piece of music.

Whereas, in humans, a restricted amount of experimental knowledge has established, for example, that septal stimulation can evoke pleasure, and orgasmic sensation, and amygdala stimulation can evoke fear and powerful uneasiness, the experiments by Nobel Laureate, Rudolph Hess, and others have shown stimulation of discrete hypothalamic sites can cause rage, snarling, hissing, eating, drinking, defecation, vomiting, micturition, and hypersexuality. This complex part of the brain is packed with nuclei. Also, Olds and colleagues have shown that implantation of electrodes in the septal area in front of the hypothalamus will cause a rat to self-stimulate thousands of times per hour in preference to food or sex. Amygdala stimulation can produce great fear. Removal of the amygdala can make animals placid and quiet, whereas, heretofore, they were aggressive. This is true also in humans. That is, there are clearly particular neural loci dictating the specificity of emotional states.

It is clear the hypothalamus is a major element in the orientation of emotional life. This is by virtue of its large projections to the cingulate, and the connections that the cingulate has to other major components of the limbic system, and to the frontal cortex.

The issue of self-awareness, at least in terms of cognizance of one's own body, has been debated in the book in relation, for example, to the fox with its foot trapped in a jawed trap, and its eating through its lower leg. Donald Griffin has asserted that a perceptively conscious grazing animal could scarcely be unaware that its companions are quietly eating or running away. A perceptively conscious animal could scarcely be unaware of its own actions such as eating and running away. Otherwise we aver the animal's mental experience is a perceptual black hole as far as its self is concerned. Self-awareness may not be unique to humans and pongids. It focuses Brentano's thoughts on intentionality, which involves a recognition of distinction between one's own thoughts, and the sensory information coming from the outside.

In the case of thirst, for example, this may come down to a value judgement. Thirst causes a strong intention to drink, which is central to consciousness, but the information from the outside may suggest a predator being present on the way to the place where it remembers there is water.

In terms of overview, it is clear that the gestalt embodied by emotion is by no means exclusively a cerebral and brainstem phenomenon. A whole spectrum of visceral, cardiovascular, respiratory, and endocrine effects evoked by it give an avalanche of sensation that feeds back upon the original cortical and basal brain processes that started the emotion. Awareness of one's own sensations becomes a dominant element in amplification of emotional state. This is conspicuously obvious with romantic love, which state has recently been neuroimaged by Zeki (1993) and others. The striatum, insula, and anterior cingulate were activated, as well as the hippocampus, hypothalamus, and ventral tegmental area.

There is a complex pattern evoked in the brain by the vision of the beloved. However, the state of sexual attraction evoked can proceed to cause penile erection and similar vascular changes in clitoris and vagina, and these processes provide powerful sensory feedback to further inflame the central state and to drive behaviour further towards the gratification with orgasm involving, *inter alia*, a localized rhythmic epileptic type phenomenon in the septum of the brain. A similar effect can be achieved by delivery of acetylcholine into the region by probes that have been placed there for therapeutic purposes. What is apparent from wide ranging studies, some of which are recounted in this book along with neuroimaging data, is that specific emotions involve a distributed system of activations and deactivations—a veritable constellation. It involves brainstem areas concerned with arousal and essential for consciousness, and the midbrain, hypothalamus, thalamus and the limbic system which latter, in turn, has protean connections to the frontal areas. Here many sensory systems converge, and from it multiple connections go to basal ganglia concerned with motor acts. Intentions are synthesized in the frontal areas. Changeux calls the frontal cortex the organ of civilization. It is concerned with calculation, anticipation and foreseeing, a role amply ratified by the famous case of Phineas Gage, who had frontal destruction and consequent profound disruption of emotional life. (Phineas Gage, a railroad worker in New England, had an accident involving a gunpowder charge that blew an iron bar through his jaw. It exited his skull in the front region of the brain. He survived for 12 years, but had profound behavioural changes. Dr Harlow, his doctor, described him as irreverent, indulging in gross profanity, without deference to his fellows, and impatient of restraint or advice conflicting with his desires. He was capricious, vacillating, and obstinate. He devised plans for future operations which were soon abandoned in favour of others.) Emotion is a particular state of consciousness, and further than that, it is the thesis of this book that it is the first embodiment of dim awareness conducive to intention, bearing, for example, on eating, drinking, breathing, reproduction, and avoiding significant core temperature changes.

Notwithstanding its cardinal importance to behaviour often determinant of the very survival of vertebrates, emotions have not been an issue that has attracted a lion's share of attention in tracts analysing consciousness. This is realistic in that processes subserving consciousness, as, for example, determined by the special senses, are much more amenable to precise analysis by neuroimaging and neurophysiological investigations. They, for example, vision, can turn on and off quickly which is advantageous for approach such as by fNMR.

Whereas a book of this size cannot pretend to present the vast body of material indubitably pertinent to its theme, it may give a general audience a perspective on the idea that particular instincts could have served the first emergence of conscious awareness.

Emotions are easily recognizable as dominant elements in human existence and behaviour, and correspondingly extend down the phylogenetic tree, as averred by Darwin in *The Expression of Emotion in Man and Animals* (1965).

At the end of the day, the overriding philosophical stance that we have adopted throughout this book comes down to the following; the mind, which has for centuries been considered as the incorporeal subject of all psychical faculties and often been severed from the body that houses it, isn't a separate entity, but quite simply and definitely what the brain does.

Glossary

In many instances, the use of a term in the text is followed immediately by a definition or explanation of function. The various parts of the brain and the various lobes of the cortex are identified in the figures. The glossary of technical terms listed here involves, in most instances, an attempt to express them as simply as possible in lay terms without too much compromise of precision.

Acetylcholine A chemical that acts as a neurotransmitter—conveys a message across a synapse.

Acetylcholine receptor A protein in the cell membrane that binds acetylcholine. It entrains events such as opening an ion channel in the membrane, or sets in train intracellular chemical processes.

Action specific energy A term used by ethologists, particularly Konrad Lorenz, to designate a build up of excitability in the brain directed to a particular behaviour.

Adrenergic Nerves that release noradrenaline, as a transmitter.

Agnatha Primitive fish without jaws, as, for example, the Lamprey.

Allocortex The older cortex, part of the limbic system of the brain, which, *inter alia*, includes olfactory cortex. It has three layers of neurons as distinct from the six layers of the neocortex.

Amniote Animals that have their embryo surrounded by a membrane: the amnion—which contains amniotic fluid. It includes all mammals, birds, and diapsid reptiles and turtles.

Amygdala An almond-shaped structure in the brain involved in emotions such as fear and aggression. It is in the front of the temporal lobe and has connections with the olfactory, limbic, and isocortex, and the basal ganglia.

Antidiuretic A hormone with actions on the kidney to cause retention of water, e.g. vasopressin.

Autonomic A division of the nervous system that innervates glands, viscera, smooth muscle, and heart and has two major components: the sympathetic and the parasympathetic.

Anosognosia Inability to acknowledge disease in oneself. Attributable to right-sided brain damage with inability, for example, to recognize that the left arm is paralysed.

Asomatognosia Inability to recognize the affected limb as one's own.

Anthropomorphic Assigning human characteristics, particularly behavioural, to animals or to ancient gods.

Basal ganglia A part of the forebrain, being large nuclei beneath the cortex, termed the caudate nucleus, globus pallidus, and putamen. They have important connections with the frontal cortex, as well as other cortical regions, and the thalamus. They are damaged in neurodegenerative diseases such as Huntington's and Parkinson's, with major disorder of voluntary movement and learned behaviour.

Behaviourism Study of animals restricted to the relationship between variations in the environment and the motor behaviour produced. The concept is aimed at eliminating the subjective from any consideration.

Brainstem General term used to designate the hindbrain and usually midbrain exclusive of the cerebellum.

Cephalopods A higher class of molluscs having a distinct head with arms or tentacles attached to it, e.g. the octopus.

Cerebellum The large lobe behind the brain hemispheres and above the hindbrain with a major role in motor processes, and more recently revealed to have a major involvement in sensory processes and emotions.

Cholinergic Neurons that release acetylcholine as a transmitter.

Cingulate cortex This is on the medial surface of the hemisphere and surrounds the corpus callosum. Deeply involved in emotional processes and also in executive functions, and in cognitive functions involving conflicting input.

Corpus callosum A very large bundle of axons (about 200 million) that cross the midline and connect the two sides of the cerebrum in placental mammals.

Diapsid designates there are two temporal openings in the skull and two bony arches.

Diencephalon The hind part of the forebrain, which includes the dorsal and ventral thalamus, hypothalamus and epithalamus (includes pineal gland).

Distance receptor Sense organs that detect stimuli at a distance from the animal: eyes, ears, nose.

Drive An inexact term suggesting a motivated tendency to act in a certain way.

Dualism The philosophic concept that the mind and the brain (matter) are independent entities.

Electroencephalogram (EEG) The variation in the waves of electrical potential recorded by electrodes attached to the scalp. In an awake tranquil person with eyes shut the changes are regular at about 10/second (alpha rhythm). When thinking, the waves are irregular. With dreamless sleep the waves are about 4/second: the delta rhythm.

Enterorhinal cortex A part of the olfactory system, which is a transitional five-layered cortex and is situated between the isocortex and the allocortical hippocampus.

ERTAS The extended reticular activation system as delineated by Baars to include the thalamic projections to the cortex.

Ethology The study of animals in their natural conditions.

Exteroceptors Sensors specialized to detect events outside the body: i.e. the eyes, ears, and nose, and also skin.

Functional magnetic resonance imaging (fMRI) A method of recording changes in blood volume and blood flow in a localized area of the brain, these altering because of the local metabolic change caused by neuronal activity. With contrast imaging based on blood oxygen level dependent (BOLD) change, the basis is that deoxygenated blood (i.e. blood that has given up its oxygen) has different magnetic properties than oxygenated blood. fMRI has better spatial resolution than positron emission tomography (PET).

Fusiform gyrus The ventral surface of the temporal lobe, which at its rear borders the occipital gyrus. A major area in colour vision function.

Gestalt An integrated whole where each individual part affects every other, the whole being more than the sum of its parts. The brain builds the whole from the pertinent perceived parts of an object, the operation of the brain being determined by both heredity and experience.

Grey Matter Brain tissue predominantly made up of neuron bodies and dendrites and appears grey. The surfaces of the hemispheres of the brain are the exemplar of grey matter.

Gyrus rectus Cortical area on the undersurface of the frontal lobe.

Hard wired The elements of behaviour patterns that are determined by heredity (i.e. genetically determined). Analogous use of a term from computer science where the program is part of the structure and not variable by the software program.

Hippocampus A medial part of the temporal lobe of the brain, which is a major centre of organization of memory.

Homeostasis The maintenance of a steady state of the internal conditions (e.g. temperature or osmotic pressure) of the body despite physical or chemical forces that would change the conditions. Claude Bernard first enunciated that the stability of the miliéu interiéur was the cardinal condition for a free life of living organisms. The process depends on inherited programmes (that is, genetically determined). They emerged by natural selection, and have great similarities across the animal kingdom, e.g. an approximate 2% rise of blood sodium concentration initiates drinking in both iguana and humans.

Hypocretin A hormone produced in the posterior and lateral hypothalamus, which stimulates feeding and arousal.

Hypothalamus A region of the brain below the thalamus and in front of the midbrain. The centre of programmes controlling homeostasis: eating and drinking and sexual reproduction and pituitary hormone secretion. The pituitary gland extends from the ventral hypothalamic surface, and through its secretions into the blood, the hypothalamus controls growth, metabolism, sexual reproduction, and reactions to stress.

Innate releasing mechanisms The genetically determined apt stimulus, which sets in train genetically determined behaviour.

Instinctual The term used to cover the inherited, i.e. genetically programmed or 'hard wired' components of behaviour. Instinctive behaviour patterns may have learning elements superimposed. (See Darwin's definition of 'instinct'—Chapter 2.)

Insula The insula is deep in the floor of the lateral sulcus and is seen when the lips of the lateral sulcus are pulled apart. It was a part of the superficial cortex but was submerged by the cortical expansion during evolution. It has several divisions and has strong connections to the anterior cingulate. It is involved, *inter alia*, in functions of the internal organs.

Intralaminar nuclei of thalamus have a crucial role in subserving consciousness. They have strong projections to the basal ganglia and also to a great deal of the neocortex. They receive cholinergic input from the brainstem and are part of the ascending reticular activating system.

Intention The aim or purpose.

Interoceptors Receptors or sensing systems that react to events or deviations from the normal within the body, e.g. core temperature, sodium concentration, blood pressure, blood CO_2, glucose concentration, and distension and pain in internal organs.

Isocortex Evolutionary more recent cortical development involving six layers of cells: e.g. the frontal, parietal, temporal, and occipital lobes.

'Knockout' (gene knockout) A molecular biological method whereby a gene is deleted from the genome, and the functional effects studied and compared with the unmodified animal (the 'wild' type).

Limbic system Structures deeply involved in emotion and memory. It includes the cingulate gyrus, insula, hippocampus, parahippocampal gyrus and subcortical structures, including amygdala, septal nuclei, and parts of the striatum and the diencephalon.

Lingual lobe Lies below the calcarine fissure of the occipital lobe at the rear of the brain, and extends round to the inferior surface of the occipital lobe and continues into the temporal lobe.

Locus ceroeleus A blue pigmented region in the pons, the axons of the neurons of which may irradiate widely in the cortex and use noradrenaline as a transmitter to arouse the cortex.

Mammillary bodies Occur bilaterally on the bottom of the hypothalamus. The fornix, which arises in the hippocampus, terminates there, and the mammillary bodies have connections with the thalamus via the mammillothalamic tract.

Medulla oblongata The rear part of the brain situated between the pons and spinal cord, where, for example, the cells controlling breathing are situated.

Mesencephalon The midbrain. It lies behind the telencephalon (the forebrain) and in front of the rhombencephalon (the hindbrain).

Micturition The physiological process of emptying the bladder: passing water or urinating.

Midbrain The part of the brain behind the thalamus and hypothalamus, and in front of the medulla: i.e. the mid-segment.

Miliéu interiéur The saline fluid medium which bathes all the cells of the body. It is the extracellular fluid of the body and carries oxygen and nutrients to the cells, and transports carbon dioxide and waste products away. Its movement depends on the pumping action of the heart. Claude Bernard made one of the landmark generalization of biology in stating that the fixité, that is, the physicochemical stability of it, was a key condition for the free life of animals.

Narcolepsy Periodic episodes involving an irresistible urge to sleep during the day.

Neocortex The most recently evolved part of the brain essential for, e.g. vision, hearing, thinking, planning, and talking.

Neuron A nerve cell having a body with a nucleus, dendrites that receive signals and usually an axon carrying nerve impulses to other cells.

Nucleus pontis oralis A part of the pons crucial to consciousness, and damage to which can induce coma.

Oesophagus The gullet, or tube conveying food and drink from the mouth to the stomach.

Operculum The lips of the lateral sulcus near its join with the central sulcus, which when pulled apart reveal the insula beneath.

Orbital gyrus Cortical area on under surface of the frontal lobe lying on the orbit, the bony structure that encloses the eye.

Pallium An embryological term meaning the covering layer of the developing cerebral hemispheres. The top or dorsal part of the telencephalon having dorsal, medial, and lateral areas.

Parabrachial nucleus Located in the dorsal pons receiving flow from the gustatory (taste) nucleus in the rear part of the medulla. It sends projections forward to the hypothalamus and amygdala, and projects also to the dorsal thalamus and the gustatory cortex.

Parahippocampus This gyrus takes up the medial part of the temporal cortex next to the hippocampus, and is a major connection between it and the neocortex. There is a convergence of many senses, including olfaction, in the parahippocampus. It plays an important part in memory.

Pavlovian conditioning Establishing an association in the brain by pairing an arbitrary stimulus: e.g. sound of a bell with an unconditioned (natural) stimulus of a genetically programmed reflex such as salivation with sight of food.

Periaqueductal gray Neuronal tissue surrounding the canal (aqueduct) between the third and fourth ventricle. Has major connections with the thalamus and anterior cingulate. *Inter alia*, it is much involved in pain mechanisms.

Perigenual The anterior cingulate cortex is wrapped around the knee or 'genu' at the front of the corpus callosum.

PET Positron emission tomography: study of activity in the living brain by injection of radioisotopes which emit positrons and permit localization of areas where blood flow is increased or decreased.

Phylogenetic tree A diagrammatic representation of the evolutionary relations between taxa. The location of the taxa depicts the relative time of their appearance in the fossil record.

Phylogeny The evolutionary history of a taxon, a taxon being a unit of a classification such as a species, a genus, or class, etc.

Plenipotentiary Exercising absolute power.

Pons The part of the brain between the medulla at its rear, and the midbrain in front. The place of location of sensory and motor nuclei of many cranial nerves, and the reticular formation, which has axon pathways both ascending and descending.

Postcentral gyrus The cortex immediately behind the central sulcus, which divides the frontal and parietal lobe. This front part of the parietal lobe receives signals from the skin and is the somatosensory cortex.

Prefrontal The anterior part of the frontal cortex.

Primary consciousness The emergence of dim awareness. The thesis of this book is, that it is the subjective component of an instinct activated by physicochemical change in the body: as, for example, thirst. In Edelman's eyes, it is the ability to construct an integrated mental scene in the present.

Primal emotion An imperious arousal compulsive of intention which has emerged during evolution because it is apt for the survival of the organism.

Putamen The caudate and lentiform nucleus are grouped as the corpus striatum. The lentiform nucleus has an internal globus pallidus and an outer putamen, which is continuous with the caudate nucleus. These basal nuclear masses are termed the basal ganglia.

Pyriform cortex A part of the olfactory system at the base of the front of the brain.

Qualia Quale (singular). The quality of a thing. The subjectivity and thus personal element of conscious experience such as the blueness of blue.

Reticular activating system (RAS) A network of neurons running up and down in the midbrain, going backward to the medulla and forward to the thalamus, and *inter alia*, responsible for programs of arousal and sleep.

Reticular nuclei of thalamus A thin sheet surrounding the thalamus, which does not project to the cerebral cortex but connects with thalamocortical and corticothalamic axons, which pass through it. It has been proposed as having a major role in the direction of attention.

Rhombencephalon The hindbrain behind (caudal) to the midbrain, and includes the cerebellum and pons, and the medulla oblongata.

Ruminants A cud chewing animal with a forestomach where bacterial and protozoal digestion of grass and foliage occurs. The term covers the bulk of the pastoral (e.g. sheep, cattle, goats) and grazing game animals (e.g. antelope, deer, and elk) of the planet.

Secondary somatosensory cortex Is at the bottom of the somatosensory cortex and is on the upper lip of the lateral fissure, which meets the central fissure at that point (see Fig. 10.4). This functional area includes the operculum.

Self-awareness Contemplation of one's own existence, being conscious of being conscious.

Semicircular canals A structure in the inner ear which is functioning to determine balance.

Septum This is situated in the medial wall of the frontal telencephalon: i.e. in the midline. It has strong connections to other limbic areas, including the amygdala and hypothalamus. Lesions in humans cause heightened emotional states and rage reactions.

Solipsism The belief that nobody really knows that anyone else is conscious. Bertrand Russell said that nobody believes it.

Somatosensory cortex The part of the cortex which receives signals from the skin. It is the posterior border of the central fissure, which divides the frontal and parietal cortex.

Split brain Cutting of the corpus callosum: the 200–300 million nerve fibres, which join the two hemispheres of the cerebrum. Done therapeutically to control severe epilepsy. The cerebrum is divided into two halves, which can be experimented on separately.

Striate cortex The primary visual cortex, which is at the back of the occipital lobe.

Striatum Also referred to as the basal ganglia which are in the ventral lateral part of the forebrain.

Stridulation A harsh shrill grating noise produced by an insect.

Subjective Having its source in the mind, i.e. belonging to the conscious life-consciousness of ones perceived states. Here the 'primal emotions' are the subjective elements of the instincts, which, *inter alia*, subserve or guard the steady state of the interior of the body.

Substantia nigra In the ventral or lower part of the tegmental area of the midbrain, and houses dopamine containing cells that project to the corpus striatum, and thus are deeply implicated in movement control.

Synapse The ending knob whereby a presynaptic axon usually contacts the dendrite of a post synaptic nerve cell. It may release a transmitter, which excites or inhibits the post synaptic cell.

Telencephalon The forebrain is composed of the telencephalon and behind it the diencephalon, which includes the thalamus, epithalamus, and hypothalamus.

Temporal lobe The part of the brain, which lies beneath the temporal bone and contains the temporal cortex on the outside, and several basal areas concerned with emotion within it.

Tegmentum Forms the dorsal portion of the brainstem except in the midbrain where the tectum is superimposed on it.

Thalamus The upper part of the diencephalon, and thus lies on top of the hypothalamus. It is a paired structure made up of many nuclei, and sends signals from the sensory systems of the body to the cortex, and receives massive feedback from the cortex.

Transitional cortex Intermediate between three-layered allocortex and six-layered isocortex.

Transmitter A chemical released at the presynaptic nerve endings, which excites or inhibits the post synaptic cell. They are mainly small molecules such as noradrenaline, acetylcholine, amino acids (e.g. glutamic acid), or purines.

V1 The first visual area of the cortex from where there is outflow to other areas designated V2, V3, V4, and V5 concerned with, for example, colour or motion detections.

Vegetative systems The various physiological organizations in the basal brain (diencephalon, mesencephalon, and hindbrain), which maintain the steady state of the internal conditions of the body. The operations are usually unconscious processes.

Ventral The area of the body that is the front of the animal (e.g. abdomen), in contrast to dorsal, which is the back of the animal.

Vermis A midline part of the cerebellum.

Vitalism The assertion that life is sustained by special forces inexplicable on the basis of principles of physics and chemistry.

White matter Brain tissue mainly made up of myelinated axons.

References

Adolph, E.F. Physiological regulation. Lancaster, Pa: Jacques Cattell Press, 1943.

Adrian, E.D. Foreword XV. In Olfaction and Taste, (C. Pfaffman ed). Rockefeller University Press, New York,1969.

Akelaitis, A.J. Studies on the corpus callosum IV Diagnostic dyspraxia in epileptics following partial and complete section of the corpus callosum. American Journal of Pyschiatry, **101**: 549–599 1945.

Alkire, M.T., Haier, R.J. and **J.H. Fallon.** Toward a unified theory of narcosis: brain imaging evidence for a thalamocortical switch as the neurophysiologic basis of anaesthetic-induced unconsciousness. *Consciousness and Cognition*, **9**: 370–386, 2000.

Anderson, B. and **McCann, S.M.** A further study of polydipsia evoked by hypothalamic stimulation in the goat. *Acta Physiologica Scandinavica*, **33**: 333, 1955.

Anderson, J.R. Self-recognition in dolphins: credible cetaceans; compromised criteria, controls and conclusions. *Consciousness and Cognition*, **4**: 239–243, 1995.

Angel, A. The **G.L. Brown** Lecture: adventures in anaesthesia. *Experimental Physiology*, **76**: 1–38, 1991.

Antognini, J.F., Buonocore, M.H., Disbrow, E.A. and **Carstens, E.** Isoflurane anesthesia blunts cerebral responses to noxious and innocuous stimuli: a fMRI study. *Life Sciences*, Pharmacol Letters, 61: 349–354, 1997.

Augustine, J.R. Circuitry and functional aspects of the insula lobe in primates including humans. *Brain Research Reviews*, **22**: 229–244, 1996.

Baars, B.J. *A Cognitive Theory of Consciousness*. Cambridge University Press, 1988.

Baars, B.J. and **Newman, J.** A Neurobiological interpretation of global workspace theory. In Revonsuo and Kamppian (eds), *Consciousness in Philosophy and Cognitive Neuroscience*. Hillsdale, NJ, 1995.

Banzett, R.B., Lansing, R.W., Brown, R., Topoulos, P., Yager, D., Steele, S.M., Loudono, B., Loring, S.H., Reid, M.B., Adams, L. and **Nations, C.S.** Air hunger from increased PCO_2 persists after complete neuromuscular block in humans. Respiratory Physiology, **80**: 1–18, 1990.

Banzett, R.B., Lansing, R.W., Evans, K.C. and **Shea, S.A.** Stimulus-response characteristics of CO_2-induced air hunger in normal subjects. *Respiration Physiology*, **103**: 19–31, 1996.

Banzett, R.B., Mulnier, H.E., Murphy, K., Rosen, S.D., Wise, R.J.S. and **Adams, L.** Breathlessness in humans activates insular cortex. *Neuroreport*, **11**: 2117–2120, 2000.

Barbeau, E. and **Poncet, M.** La dyspraxie diagonistique dans les lésions antérieures et postérieures du corps calleux. Revue de Neuropsychologie, **11**: 241–256, 2001.

Barbeau, E. and **Poncet, M.** La dyspraxie diagonistique dans les lésions antérieures et postérieures du corps calleux. *Revue de Neuropsychologie*, **11**: 241–256, 2001.

Bateson, P. Do animals feel pain? *New Scientist*, **134**: 30, 1992.

Bennett, M. R. *The Idea of Consciousness. Synpases and the Mind.* Harwood Academic Publishers, Amsterdam, 1997.

Bernard, C. *An Introduction to the Study of Experimental Medicine*. Dover Publications Inc., New York, 1957.

Biederman, G.B. and Davey, V.A. Social learning in invertebrates. Science, **259**: 1627–1628, 1993.

Blair-West, J.R., Denton, D.A., McKinley, M.J., Radden, B.G., Ramshaw, E.H. and Wark, J.D. Behavioural and tissue responses to severe phosphate depletion in cattle. American Journal of Physiology, **263**: R656–663, 1992.

Blok, B.F.M., Willemsen, A.T. and Holstege, G. A PET study on brain control of micturition in humans. *Brain*, **120**: 111–121, 1997.

Bonhomme, V., Fiset, P., Meuret, P., Backman, S., Plourde, G., Paus, T., Bushnell, M.C. and Evans, A.C. Propofol anesthesia and cerebral blood flow changes elicited by vibrotactile stimulation: a positron emission tomography study. *Journal of Neurophysiology*, **85**: 1299–1308, 2001.

Bradshaw, S.D. Volume regulation in desert reptiles and its control by pituitary and adrenal hormones. In C. Barker Jorgenson, E. Schadhauge (eds) Osmotic and Volume Regulation. Proceedings of Alfred Benzon Symposium XI, Munksgaard, Copenhagen, p55, 1978.

Brannan, S., Liotti, M., Egan, G., Shade, R., Madden, L., Robbillard, R., Abplanalp, B., Stofer, K., Denton, D. and Fox, P.T. Neuroimaging of cerebral activations and deactivations associated with hypercapnia and hunger for air. *Proceedings of the National Academy of Sciences USA*, **98**: 2029–2034, 2001.

Bridgman, P.W. *The Logic of Modern Physics*. The Macmillan Company, New York, 1927.

Bromm, B. Brain images of pain. *News in Physiological Sciences*, **16**: 244, 2001.

Brown, C. Not just a pretty face in animal minds – clever fish. New Scientist, 182: 42–43, June 2004.

Bullock, T.H. After thoughts on animal minds. In: Griffin, D.R. (ed.) *Animal Mind–Human Mind*. Dahlem Konferenzen. Springer Verlag, Berlin, 1982, pp. 407–414.

Bullock, T.J. and Basar, E. Comparison of ongoing compound field potentials in the brains of invertebrates and vertebrates. Brain Research, **472**: 57–75, 1988.

Burghardt, G.M. Cognitive ethology and critical anthropomorphism: a snake with two heads and hognose snakes that play dead. In: Ristau, C.A. (ed.) *Cognitive Ethology. The Minds of Other Animals. Essays in Honor of Donald R. Griffin*. Lawrence Erlbaum, Hillsdale, NJ, 1991.

Bush, G., Lau, P. and Posner, M.I. Cognitive and emotional influences in anterior cingulate cortex. *Trends in Cognitive Science*, **4**: 216, 2000.

Butler, A. and Hodos, W. *Comparative Vertebrate Neuroanatomy. Evolution and Adaptation*. Wiley Liss, Hoboker, New Jersey 2005 (1st edition 1996).

Butler, A.B. and Cotterill, R.M.J. Mammalian and avian neuroanatomy and the questions of consciousness in birds. Biological Bulletin, (in press 2006)

Butler, A.B., Manger, P.R., Lindahl, B.I.B. and Arhem, P. Evolution of the neural basis of consciousness : a bird-mammal comparison. Bioessays, **27**: 923–936, 2005.

Cannon, W.B. *Proceedings of the Royal Society* (London), **90**: 283, 1919.

Changeux, J.-P. *Neuronal Man—The Biology of Mind*. Oxford University Press, 1985.

Changeux, J.-P. *L'Homme de Vérité*. Editions Odile Jacob, Paris 2002, and Harvard University Press, 2003.

Changeux, J.-P. and Connes, A. *Conversation on Mind, Matter and Mathematics*. Princeton University Press, 1995.

Coghill, R.C., Talbot, J.D., Evans, A.C., Meyer, E., Gjedde, A., Bushnell, M.C. and Duncan, G.H. Distributed processing of pain and vibration by the human brain. *Journal of Neuroscience*, **14**: 4095–4108, 1994.

Colebatch, J.G., Adams, L., Murphy, K., Martin, A.J., Lammertsma, Tochon-Danguy, H.J., Clark, J.L., Friston, K.J. and Guz, A. Regional cerebral blood flow during volitional breathing in man. *Journal of Physiology*, **443**: 91–103, 1991.

Craig, A.D. A new view of pain as a homeostatic emotion. *Trends in Neurosciences*, **26**: 303–307, 2003.

Craig, A.D., Chen, K., Bandy, D. and Reiman, E.M. Thermosensory activation of insular cortext. *Nature Neuroscience*, **3**: 184–190, 2000.

Craig, W. Appetite and aversions as constituents of instincts. *Biological Bulletin*, **2**: 91–107, 1918.

Crick, F. Function of the thalamic reticular complex: the searchlight hypothesis. *Proceedings of the National Academy of Sciences USA*, **81**: 4586–4590, 1984.

Crick, F. *The Astonishing Hypothesis: The Scientific Search for the Soul*. Simon & Schuster, London, 1994.

Crick, F. Interviewed by Margaret Wertheim. *New York Times* 13 April, 2004.

Crick, F. and Koch, C. A framework for consciousness. *Nature Neuroscience*, **6**: 119–126, 2003.

Crick, F.C. and Koch, C. Consciousness and Neuroscience. Cerebral Cortex, **8**: 97–107, 1998.

Damasio, A.R. *Descartes' Error*. Avon Books, New York, 1994.

Damasio, A.R. How the brain creates the mind. *Scientific American*, **December**: 74–79, 1999a.

Damasio, A.R., Grabowski, T.J., Bechara, A., Damasio, H., Ponto, L.I.B., Ponto, J.P. and Hichura, R.D. Subcortical and cortical brain activity during the feeling of self-generated emotions. Nature Neuroscience, **3**: 1049–1056, 2000.

Damasio, A. *The Feeling of What Happens. Body, Emotion and the Making of Consciousness*. Random House, London, 1999b.

Darwin, C. On the Origin of Species, John Murray, London, 1859.

Darwin, C. *The Expression of the Emotions in Man and Animals*. University of Chicago Press, Chicago, 1965.

Davidson, R.J. and Irwin, W. The functional neuroanatomy of emotion and affective style. *Trends in Cognitive Science*, **3**: 11–21, 1999.

Dawes, J., Fernandes, J. and Robertson, J.D. *Octopus vulgaris* can learn by visual observation. American Association of Anatomists 106th Meeting. *Anatomical Record*, Suppl. 1B, 1993.

Dawkins, M.S. Animal minds and animal emotions. *American Zoologist*, **40**: 883–888, 2000.

Dehaene, S., Kerszberg, M. and Changeux, J.-P. A neuronal model of a global workspace in effortful cognitive tasks. *Proceedings of the National Academy of Sciences, USA*, **95**: 14529–14534, 1998.

Denton, D.A. *The Hunger for Salt: An anthropological, physiological and medical analysis* Springer-Verlag, London, 1983.

Denton, D.A. The Pinnacle of Life : Consciousness and self-awareness in humans and animals. 1993, Allen & Unwin, Sydney; 1994, Harper Collins, San Francisco, Flammarion, Paris, and English Language Publishing Company, Japan.

Denton, D.A., McKinley, M.J. and Weisinger, R.S. Hypothalamic integration of body fluid regulation. *Proceedings of the National Academy of Sciences USA*, **93**, 7397–7404, 1996.

Denton, D.A., Shade, R., Zamarippa, F., Egan, G., Blair–West, J., McKinley, M. and Fox, P. The correlation of regional cerebral blood flow (rCBF) and change of plasma sodium concentration during genesis and satiation of thirst. *Proceedings of the National Academy of Sciences USA*, **96**: 2532–2537, 1999a.

Denton, D.A., Shade, R., Zamarippa, F., Egan, G., Blair-West, J., McKinley, M., Lancaster, J. and Fox, P. Neuroimaging of genesis and satiation of thirst: an interoceptor driven theory of origins of primary consciousness. *Proceedings of the National Academy of Sciences USA*, **96**: 5304–5309, 1999b.

Derbyshire, S.W.G. A Systemic review of neuroimaging data during visceral stimulation. *American Journal of Gastroenterology*, **98**, 13–20, 2003.

Devinsky, O., Morrell, M.J. and Vogt, B.A. Contributions of anterior cingulate cortex to behaviour. *Brain*, **118**: 279–306, 1995.

Dolan, R.J. Emotion, cognition and behaviour. *Science*, **298**: 119–122, 2002.

Eccles, J.C. (ed) Brain and Conscious Experience. Study Week of the Pontifical Academy of Science, Springer Verlag, Berlin, 1966.

Eccles, J. See Denton D.A., *The Pinnacle of Life—consciousness and self-awareness in humans and animals*. Flammarion, Paris, 1995, Harper Collins 1994. Allen and Unwin 1993.

Eckhorn, R., Bauer, R., Jordan, W., Brosch, M., Kruse, W., Munk, M. and Reitboeck, H.J. Coherent oscillations: a mechanism of feature linking in the visual cortex? *Biological Cybernetics*, **60**: 121–130, 1988.

Edelman, G.M. *Neural Darwinism: The Theory of Neuronal Group Selection*. Basic Books, New York, 1987.

Edelman, G.M. *The Remembered Present: a biological theory of consciousness*. Basic Books, New York, 1989.

Edelman, G.M. *Bright Air, Brilliant Fire: on the matter of the mind*. Basic Books, New York, 1992.

Edelman, G.M. Building a picture of the brain. *Daedalus (Journal of the American Academy of Arts and Sciences)*, **127**: 37–69, 1998.

Edelman, G.M. Naturalizing consciousness: a theoretical framework. *Proceedings of the National Academy of Sciences USA*, **100**: 5520–5524, 2003.

Edelman, G.M. and Tononi, G. *A Universe of Consciousness: How Matter Becomes Imagination*. Basic Books, New York, 2000.

Egan, G., Silk, T., Zamarripa, F., Williams, J., Federico, P., Cunnington, R., Carabott, L., Blair-West, J., Shade, R., McKinley, M., Farrell, M., Lancaster, J., Fox, P., and Denton, D. Neural correlates of the emergence of consciousness of thirst. *Proceedings of the National Academy of Sciences USA*, **100**: 15241–15246, 2003.

Engelage, J. and Bischof, H.-J. The organization of the tectofugal pathway in birds. a comparative review. In: Zeigler, H.P. and Bischof, H.-J. (eds). *Vision, Brain and Behavior in Bird*. The MIT Press, Cambridge, MA, 1993, pp. 137–158.

Evans, K.C., Banzett, R.B., Adams, L., McKay, L., Frackowiak, R.S. and Corfield, D.R. BOLD fMRI identifies limbic, paralimbic and cerebellar activations during air hunger. *Journal of Neurophysiology*, **88**: 1500–1511, 2002.

Fioritto, G. and Scotto, P. Observational learning in *Octopus vulgaris*. *Science*, **256**: 545–547, 1992.

Fiset, P., Paus, T., Daloze, T., Plourde, G., Meuret, P., Bonhomme, V., Haji-Ali, N., Backman, S.B. and Evans, A.C. Brain mechanisms of propofol-induced loss of consciousness in humans: a positron emission tomographic study. *Journal of Neuroscience*, **19**: 5506–5513, 1999.

Fitzsimons, J. *Physiology of Thirst and Sodium Appetite*. Cambridge University Press, 1979.

Fitzsimons, J.T. Angiotensin, thirst, and sodium appetite. *Physiological Reviews*, **78**: 583–686, 1998.

Franks, N.P. and Lieb, W.R. Molecular and cellular mechanisms of general anaesthesia. *Nature*, **367**: 607–614, 1994.

Gallup, G.G. Jnr. Chimpanzees: self-recognition. *Science*, **167**: 86–87, 1970.

Gallup, G.G. Jnr. Towards an operational definition of self-awareness. In: Tuttle, R.H. (ed.), *Socio-Ecology and Psychology of Primates*. Mouton & Co, The Hague, 1975, pp. 309–341.

Gallup, G.G. Jnr. Self-recognition in primates: a comparative approach to the bidirectional properties of consciousness. *American Psychologist*, 329, 1977.

Gallup, G.G. Jnr. Toward a comparative psychology of mind. In: Mellgren, R.L. (ed.), *Animal Cognition and Behavior*. North-Holland, Amsterdam, 1983, pp. 473–510.

Gallup, G.G. Jnr. Self-awarness. In: Mitchell, G. and Erwin, J. (eds), *Comparative Primate Biology, Behavior, Cognition and Motivation*, Vol. 2, Part B. Liss, New York, 1987, pp. 3–16.

Gallup, G.G. Jnr. Toward a comparative psychology of self-awareness: species limitations and cognitive consequences. In: Goethals, G.R. and Strauss, J. (eds), *The Self: An Interdisciplinary Approach*. Springer-Verlag, New York, 1991, pp. 121–135.

Gandevia, S.C., Killean, K., McKanne, D.R., Crawford, M., Allen, G.M., Gorman, R.B. and Hales, J.P. Respiratory sensations, cardiovascular control, Kinaesthia and transcranial stimulation during paralysis in humans. Journal of Physiology, **470**: 85–107, 1993.

Gazzaniga, M.S. The Social Brain. Discovering the Networks of the Mind. Basic Books, New York 1985.

George, M.S., Ketter, T., Parekh, A., Priti, I, Horwitz, B. Herscovitch, P. and Post, R.M. Brain activity during transient sadness and happiness in healthy women. *American Journal of Psychiatry*, **152**(3): 341–351, 1995.

Gillette, R. The Molluscan Nervous System. Comparative Animal Psychology – Neural and Integrative Physiology, C. Prosser (ed), Wiley, New York, 1991.

Gould, J.L. and Gould, C.G. Invertebrate intelligence. In Hoage, R.J. and Goldman, L. (eds), *Animal Intelligence. Insights into the Animal Mind*. Smithsonian Institution Press, Washington DC, 1986, pp. 21–36.

Granon, S., Faure, P. and Changeux, J.-P. Executive and social behaviors under nicotinic receptor regulation. *Proceedings of the National Academy of Sciences USA*, **100**: 9596–9601, 2003.

Gray, C.M. and Singer, W. Stimulus-specific neuronal oscillations in orientation columns of cat visual cortex. *Proceedings of the National Academy of Sciences USA*, **86**: 1698–1702, 1989.

Gray, C.M., König, P., Engel, A.K. and Singer, W. Oscillatory responses in cat visual cortex exhibit inter-columnar synchronization which reflects global stimulus properties. *Nature*, **338**: 334–337, 1989.

Griffin, D.R. *Animal Minds*. University of Chicago Press, 1992.

Griffin, D.R. Scientific approaches to animal consciousness. *American Zoology*, **4**: 889–892, 2000.

Grossman, R.G. Are current concepts and methods in neuroscience adequate for studying the neural basis of consciousness and mental activity. In Pinsker, H.M. and Willis Jr, W.D. (eds), *Information Processing in the Nervous System*. Raven Press, New York, 1980, pp. 331.

Guz, A. Brain, breathing and breathlessness. *Respiration Physiology*, **109**: 197–204, 1997.

Hauser, M.D., Kralik, J., Botto-MaHan, C., Garrett, M. and Oser, J. Self-recognition in primates: phylogeny and the salience of species—typical features. *Proceedings of the National Academy of Sciences USA*, **92**: 10811–10814, 1995.

Heath, R.G. Pleasure and brain activity in man. *Journal of Nervous and Mental Disease*, **54**: 3, 1972.

Hebb, D.O. The Organization of Behaviour, Wiley, New York, 1949.

Herrnstein, R.J. and Loveland, D.H. Complex visual concept in the pigeon. *Science*, **146**: 549, 1964.

Herrnstein, R.J., Loveland, D.H. and Cable, C. Natural concepts in pigeons. *Journal of Experimental Psychology Animal Behaviour Processes*, **2**: 285, 1976.

Higuchi, H. Bait fishing by the green backed heron *Ardeola striata* in Japan. *Ibis*, **128**: 285–290, 1986.

Hobson, J.A. The Dreaming Brain. Basic Books Inc., New York, 1988.

Hodos, W. and Campbell, C.B.G. Evolutionary scales and comparative studies of cognition. In: Kesner, R. and Olton, D. (eds), *Animal Cognition*. Erlbaum, Hillsdale, NJ, 1990, pp. 1–21.

Holstege, G., Georgiadis, J.R., Paans, A.M.J., Meiners, L.C., van der Graaf, F.H.C.E. and Reinders, A.A.T.S. Brain activation during human male ejaculation. *Journal of Neuroscience*, **23**: 9185–9193, 2003.

Horgan, D. *The Undiscovered Mind: How the brain defies explanation*. Weidenfield & Nicholson, 1999.

Hubel, D.H. and Wiesel, T.N. The Ferrier Lecture: Functional architecture of the *Macaque* monkey visual cortex. *Proceedings of the Royal Society (London) B*, **198**: 1, 1997.

Huxley, T.H. On Descartes' discourse touching the method of using one's reason rightly and of seeking scientific truth. In: *Method and Results*. D. Appleton and Co., New York, pp. 166–198, 1898a.

Huxley, T.H. On the hypothesis that animals are automata and its history. In: *Methods and Results*. D. Appleton and Co., New York, pp. 199–240, 1898b.

Izzard, C.E. *Human Emotions*. Plenum Press, New York, 1977.

James, W. *The Principles of Psychology* (1890). American Science Series (2 Vols). Henry Holt and Co., New York, 1918.

Jones, P.G., Rosser, S.J. and Bulloch, A.G.M. Glutamate suppression of feeding and the underlying output of effector neurons in *Helisoma*. *Brain Research*, **437**: 56–68, 1987.

Jouvet, M. *Le Sommeil et le Rêve*. Editions Odile Jacob, 1992.

Kandel, E.R., Schwartz, J.H. and Jessell, T.M. *Principles of Neural Science*, 3rd edn. Elsevier, New York, 1991.

Keenan, J.P., Nelson, A., O'Connor, M. and Paseual-Leone, A. Self-recognition and the right hemisphere. *Nature*, **409**: 305, 2001.

Kenny, A.J.P. In: The Development of the Mind, A.J.P. Kenny, H.C. Longuet-Higgins, J.R. Lucas and C.H. Waddington (ed) Edinburgh University Press, 1973.

Killdaff, T.S. and Peyron, C. The hypocretin/orexin ligand receptor system: implications for sleep and sleep disorders. *Trends in cognition science*, **23**: 359–365, 2000.

Kinomura, S., Larsson, J., Gulyas, B. and Roland, P.E. Activation by attention of the human reticular formation and thalamic intralaminar nuclei. *Science*, **271**: 512–515, 1996.

Kitchen, A., Denton, D.A. and Brent, L. Self-recognition and abstraction abilities in the common chimpanzee studied with distorting mirrors. *Proceedings of the National Academy of Sciences USA*, **93**: 7405–7408, 1996.

Kleinginna, P.R.Jr. and Kleinginna, A.M. A categorized list of emotion definitions, with suggestions for a consensual definition. *Motivation & Emotion*, **5**: 345–379, 1981.

Koch, C. *The Quest for Consciousness*. Roberts & Co. Publishers, Boulder, CO, 2004.

Laland, K.N., Brown, C. and Krause, J. Learning in fishes: from three-second memory to culture. *Fish and Fisheries*, **4**, 199–202, 2004.

LeDoux, J. *The Emotional Brain. The Myserious Underpinnings of Emotional Life.* Touchstone (Simon & Schuster Inc.), New York, 1998.

LeDoux, J.E. and Hirst, W. *Mind andF Brain*. Cambridge University Press, 1986.

Levy, L.M., Henkin, R.L., Lin, C.S., Finley, A. and Schellinger, D. Taste memory induces brain activation as revealed by functional MRI. *Journal of Computer Assisted Tomography*, **23**: 499–505, 1999a.

Levy, L.M., Henkin, R.I., Lin, C.S. and Hutter, A. Odor memory induces brain activation as measured by functional MRI. *Journal of Computer Assisted Tomography*, **23**: 487–498, 1999b.

Lindauer, M. Communication among Social Bees (2nd edition). Harvard University Press, Cambridge, Mass., 1971

Liotti, M. and Mayberg, H.S. The role of functional neuroimaging in the neuropsychology of depression. *Journal of Clinical and Experimental Neuropsychology*, **23**: 121–136, 2001.

Liotti, M., Mayberg, H.S., Brannan S.K., McGinnis, S., Jerabek, P. and Fox, P.T. Differential limbic–cortical correlates of sadness and anxiety in health subjects: implications for affective disorders. *Biological Psychiatry*, **48**: 30–42, 2000.

Liotti, M., Brannan, S., Egan, G., Shade, R., Madden, L., Abplanalp, B., Robillard, R., Lancaster, J., Zamarripa, F.E., Fox, P.T. and Denton, D. Brain responses associated with consciousness of breathlessness (air hunger). *Proceedings of the National Academy of Sciences USA*, **99**: 2035–2040, 2001.

Lorenz, K.Z. The comparative method in studying innate behaviour patterns. In: *Physiological Mechanisms in Animal Behaviour—Symposia of Society of Experimental Biology*. Cambridge University Press, 1950.

Loveland, K.A. Self-recognition in the bottlenose dolphin: ecological considerations. *Consciousness and Cognition*, **4**: 254–257, 1995.

Lovell, H.B. Baiting of fish by a Green Heron. *Wilson Bulletin*, **70**(3): 280–281, 1958.

Maldonado, H. The visual attack learning system in *Octopus Vulgaris*. *Journal of Theoretical Biology*, **5**: 470-488, 1963.

Maquet, P., Degueldre, C., Delfiore, G., Aerts, J., Péters, J.-M., Luxen, A. and Franck, G. Functional neuroanatomy of human slow wave sleep. *Journal of Neuroscience*, **17**: 2807–2812, 1997.

Maquet, P., Péters, J.-M., Aerts, J., Delfiore, G., Degueldre, C., Luxen, A., and Franck, G. Functional neuroanatomy of human rapid-eye movement sleep and dreaming. *Nature*, **383**: 163–166, 1996.

Marten, K. and Psarakos, S. Using self-view television to distinguish between self-examination and social behavior in the bottlenose dolphin (*Tursiops truncatus*). *Consciousness and Cognition*, 4: 205–224, 1995.

Mason, W.A. Windows on other minds. *Science*, 194: 930–931, 1976.

Mayberg, H.S. Frontal lobe dysfunction in secondary depression. *Journal of Neuropsychiatry and Clinical Neurosciences*, 6: 428–442, 1994.

Mayberg, H.S. Limbic-cortical dysregulation: a proposed model of depression. *Journal of Neuropsychiatry*, 9: 471–481, 1997.

Mayberg, H.S., Liotti, M, Brannan, S., McGinis, S., Mahurin, R.K., Jerabek, P.A., Silva, J.A., Tekell, J.L., Martin, C.C., Lancaster, J.L. and Fox, P.T. Reciprocal limbic-cortical function and negative mood: converging PET findings in depression and normal sadness. *American Journal of Psychiatry*, 156: 675–682, 1999.

McDougall, W. *An Outline of Psychology*. Methuen Publishers, London, 1923.

Miklos, G.L.G. The evolution and modification of brains and sensory systems. *Daedalus (Journal of the American Academy of Arts and Sciences)*, 127: 197–216, 1998.

Mitchell, R.W. Mental models of mirror-self-recognition: two theories. *New Ideas in Psychology*, 11: 295–325, 1993.

Monod, J. *Chance and Necessity*. Collins Publishers, London, 1972.

Mountcastle, V.B. Modality and topographic properties of single neurones of cats' somatic sensory cortex. *Journal of Neurophysiology*, 20: 408, 1957.

Mountcastle, V.B. (ed.) Sleep, wakefulness, and the conscious state: intrinsic regulatory mechanisms of the brain. In: *Medical Physiology*. CV Mosby, St Louis, 1980.

Newman, J. Putting the puzzle together, Part I: towards a general theory of the neural correlates of consciousness. *Journal of Consciousness Studies*, 4: 47–66, 1997a.

Newman, J. Putting the puzzle together, Part II: towards a general theory of the neural correlates of consciousness. *Journal of Consciousness Studies*, 4(2): 100–121, 1997b.

Newman, J. and Baars, B.J. A neural attentional model for access to consciousness: a global workspace perspective. *Concepts in Neuroscience*, 4: 255–290, 1993.

Nitz, D.A., van Swinderen, B., Tononi, G. and Greenspan, R.J. Electrophysiological correlates of rest and activity in *Drosophila melanogaster*. *Current Biology*, 12: 1934–1940, 2002.

Oakley, K.P. Skill as a Human Possession, In History of Technology Vol.1, C. Singer (ed), Oxford University Press (London) 1954.

Oatley, K. and Jenkins, J. *Understanding Emotions*. Blackwell Publishing, Oxford, 1996.

Overmier, J.B. and Hollis, K.L. Fish in the think tank: learning, memory and integrated behavior. In: Kesner, R.P. and Olton, D.S. (eds). *Neurobiology of Comparative Cognition*, Lawrence Erlbaum, Hillsdale, NJ, 1990.

Panksepp, J. *Affective Neuroscience. The Foundations of Human and Animal Emotions*. Oxford University Press Inc., New York, 1998.

Papez, J.W. A proposed mechanism of emotion. *Archives of Neurology & Psychiatry*, 38: 725–743, 1937.

Parsons, L.M., Denton, D., Egan, G., McKinley, M., Shade, R., Lancaster, J. and Fox, P.T. Neuroimaging evidence implicating cerebellum in support of sensory/cognitive processes associated with thirst. *Proceedings of the National Academy of Sciences USA*, 97: 2332–2336, 2000.

Parsons, L.M., Egan, E., Liotti, M., Brannan, S., Denton, D., Shade, R., Robillard, R., Madden, L., Abplanalp, B. and Fox, P.T. Neuroimaging evidence implicating cerebellum in the experience of hypercapnia and hunger for air. *Proceedings of the National Academy of Sciences USA*, 99: 2041–2046, 2001.

Pashler, H., Luck, S.J., Hillyard, S.A., Mangun, G.R., O'Brien, S. and Gazzaniga, M.S. Sequential operating of disconnected cerebral hemispheres in split brain patients. *Neuro-Report*, 5: 2381–2384, 1994.

Peiffer, C., Proline, J.B, Thivardl-Aubiert, M. and Samson, Y. Neural substrates for the perception of acutely induced dyspnoea. *American Journal of Respiratory and Critical Care Medicine*, 163: 951–957, 2001.

Peyron, R., Laurent, B. and Garcia Larrea, L. Functional imaging of brain response to pain. A review and meta-analysis. *Neurophysiology Clin.*, 5: 263–288, 2000.

Pitts, G.C. An evolutionary approach to pain. *Perspectives in Biology and Medicine*, 37: 275, 1994.

Plum, F., Schiff, N., Ribrary, U. and Llinás, R. Coordinated expression in chronically unconscious persons. *Philosophical Transactions of the Royal Society London*, 353: 1929–1933, 1998.

Plutchik, R. Emotion: A psychoevolutionary synthesis. Harper & Row, New York, 1980.

Powers, A.S. Brain mechanisms of learning in reptiles. In: Kesner, R.P. and Olton, D.S. (eds), *Neurobiology of Comparative Cognition*. Lawrence Erlbaum, Hillsdale, NJ, 1990.

Proust, M. *Remembrance of Things Past*. Translated by C.K. Scott Moncrieff and Terence Kilmartin. Penguin Books, London, 1983.

Rainville, P., Duncan, G.H., Price, D.D., Carrier, B. and Bushnell, M.C. Pain affect encoded in human anterior cingulate but not somatosensory cortex. *Science*, 277: 968–971, 1997.

Redmond, I. The salt-mining elephants of Mt Elgon. *Wildlife*, **August** 1982.

Redmond, I. Underground elephants. Animal kingdom. *New York Zoological Society Magazine*, December 1984–January 1985.

Redmond, I. Report on Ivory Poaching in the Mount Elgon National Park. July 1987.

Redmond, I. Elephant family values. In: Taylor, V.I. and Dunstone, N. (eds), *The Exploitation of Mammal Populations*. Chapman & Hall, London, 1996.

Reiss, D. and Marino, L. Mirror self-recognition in the bottlenose dolphin: a case of cognitive convergence. *Proceedings of the National Academy of Sciences USA*, 98: 5937–5942, 2001.

Richter, C.P. The Psychobiology of Curt Richter (E. Blass ed.) York Press, Baltimore, 1976.

Robinson, B.W. and Mishkin, M. Alimentary responses to forebrain stimulation in monkeys. *Experimental Brain Research*, 4: 330–366, 1968.

Roland, P.E., Eriksson, L. Stone-Elander, S. and Widen, L. Does mental activity change the oxidative metabolism of the brain? *Journal of Neuroscience*, 7(8): 2373–2389, 1987.

Rolls, E.T. *The Brain and Emotions*. Oxford University Press, 1999.

Rolls, E.T. The orbitofrontal cortex and reward. *Cerebral Cortex*, 10: 284–294, 2000.

Rose, J.D. The neurobehavioural nature of fishes and the question of awareness and pain. *Reviews and Fisheries Science*, 10: 1–38, 2002.

Rose, M. Gyrus Limbicus anterior und regio retrosplenialis (Cortex holoprotoptychos quinqestratificus). Vergleichende Architektonik bei Tier und Mensch. *Journal of Psychology and Neurology*, 35: 65–173, 1927.

Sanders, .K.F. and **Young, J.Z.** Learning and other functions of the higher nervous centres of *Sepia, Journal of Neurophysiology*, **3**: 501–525, 1940.

Schmahmann, J.D. and **Sherman, J.C.** The cerebellar cognitive affective syndrome. *Brain*, **121**: 561–579, 1998.

Schmidt-Nielsen, K. *Desert Animals: physiological problems of heat and water.* Oxford University Press, 1964.

Searle, J.R. *Intentionality: an essay in the philosophy of mind.* Cambridge University Press, Cambridge, 1983.

Searle, J.R. *Minds, Brains and Science.* The 1984 Reith Lectures, London, British Broadcasting Corporation. Penguin Books, 1989; Harvard University Press, Cambridge, MA, 1985.

Searle, J.R. *The Mystery of Consciousness*, Granta Books (London), 1997.

Searle, J.R. *The Rediscovery of the Mind.* MIT Press, Cambridge, Mass., 1992.

Searle, J.R. *The Problem of Consciousness.* http:www.u.arizona.edu/~chalmers/online.html

Seitz, R.J. and **Roland, P.E.** Learning of sequential finger movements in man: a combined kinematic and Positron Emission Tomography (PET) study. *European Journal of Neuroscience*, **4**: 154–165, 1992.

Sewards, T.V. and **Sewards, M.A.** The awareness of thirst: Proposed neural correlates. *Consciousness and Cognition*, **9**: 463–487, 2000.

Shaw, P.J., Cirelli, C., Greenspan, R.J. and **Tononi, G.** Correlates of sleep and waking in *Drosophila melanogaster. Science*, **287**: 1834–1837, 2000.

Singer, W. Neural synchrony : a versatile code for the definition of relations. *Neuron*, **24**: 49-65, 1999.

Skinner, B.F. *Beyond Freedom and Dignity.* Kopf, New York, 1971, p. 199.

Smith, H.W. The biology of consciousness. In: Brooks, C.McC. and Cranefield, P. (eds), *The Historical Development of Physiological Thought.* The Hafner Publishing Co., New York, 1959, pp. 109–136.

Sperry, R.W. Lateral specialization in the surgically separated hemispheres. In Schmitt, F.O. *et al.* (eds), *The Neurosciences.* Third Study Program, MIT Press, Cambridge, MA, p. 5, 1974.

Stellar, E. Drive and motivation. In: Field, J., Mazour, H.W. and Hall, V.E. (eds), *Handbook of Physiology: Neurophysiology*, Vol. 3. American Physiological Society, Washington, DC, 1960.

Steriade, M. *Thalamus, Encyclopedia of Neuroscience*, Vol. II, Adelman, G. (ed.). Birkhauser Boston Inc., Boston, 1987, pp. 1204–1208.

Suboski, M.D., Muir, D. and Hall, D. Social learning in invertebrates. *Science*, **259**: 1629, 1993

Sutcliffe, A.J. Caves of East Africa Rift Valley. *Transactions of the Cave Research Group of Great Britain*, **15**: 41, 1973.

Tanaka, Y., Iwasa, H. and **Yoshida, M.** Diagnostic dyspraxia: case report and movement-related potentials. *Neurology*, **40**: 657–661, 1990.

Tataranni, P.A., Gautier, J.-F., Chen, K., Ueckler, A., Bandy, D., Salbe, A.D., Pratley, R.E., Lawson, M., Reiman, E.M. and **Ravussin, E.** Neuroanatomical correlates of hunger and satiation in humans using positron emission tomography. *Proceedings of the National Academy of Sciences USA*, **96**: 4569–4574, 1999.

Thompson, W.L. and Kosslyn, S.M. Neural systems activated during visual mental imagery. In *Brain Mapping The Systems* (A.W. Toga & J.C. Mazziotta eds) 535–560, Academic Press, San Diego, 2000.

Thorpe, W.H. Ethology and consciousness. In: Eccles, J.C. (ed.), *Brain and Conscious Experience*. Springer-Verlag, Berlin, 1966.

Tinbergen, N. *The Study of Instinct*. Oxford University Press, 1951.

Tolstoy, L. *War and Peace*. Penguin Classics, 1957.

Tononi, G. and Edelman, G.M. Consciousness and complexity. *Science*, **282**: 1846–1850, 1998.

Trotter, W. *Instincts of the Herd in Peace and War*. T. Fisher Unwin Ltd, London, 1922.

Vogt, B.A. and Gabriel, M. *Neurobiology of Cingulate Cortex and Limbic Thalamus*. Birkhauser, Boston, MA, 1993.

Walker, S. *Animal Thought*. Routledge & Kegan Paul, London, 1983.

Watson, J.B. Psychology as the behaviourist views it. *Pyschology Review*, **20**: 158, 1913.

Weir, J.S. Spatial distribution of elephants in an African national park in relation to environmental sodium. *Oikos*, **23**: 1–3, 1972.

Whitman, C.O. *Animal Behaviour*. Biology Lectures of the Marine Biological Laboratory, Woods Hole, MA, 1899.

Woolf, V. *The Common Reader* (second series). Hogarth Press, London, 1953.

Young, J.Z. *A Model of the Brain*. Oxford University Press, London, 1964.

Young, J.Z. *Philosophy and the Brain*. Oxford University Press, 1986.

Zaidel, D.W. A view of the world from a split brain perspective. In: Critchley, E.M.R. (ed.), *The Neurological Boundaries of Reality*. Farrand Press, London, 1994, pp. 161–174.

Zeki, S. *A Vision of the Brain*. Blackwell Scientific Publications, Oxford, 1993.

Author Index

Subject Index